Making Use of Guidelines in Clinical Practice

Edited by

Allen Hutchinson
and
Richard Baker

Foreword by

Sir Donald Irvine

RADCLIFFE MEDICAL PRESS

Radcliffe Medical Press Ltd
18 Marcham Road, Abingdon, Oxon OX14 1AA

British Library Cataloguing in Publication Data
A catalogue record for this book is available from the British Library.

ISBN 1 85775 088 8

Typeset by Joshua Associates Ltd, Oxford
Printed and bound by Biddles Ltd, Guildford and King's Lynn

Contents

Foreword

Medicine is now well into the era of explicit professional and clinical standards. Clinical guidelines flow from the drive to secure clinical decision making which is based on the best research evidence available and which is, therefore, as demonstrably effective as possible. It is clearly in patients' interests that doctors apply good practice as consistently as they can, and that inappropriate variation is eliminated.

In using clinical guidelines, I believe that clinicians must retain the freedom to decide with their individual patients what is best in the circumstances, since all patients are different. The important thing, in the exercise of that clinical judgement, is that doctors must always be prepared to justify their decisions. Neither arbitrariness at one end of the scale of clinical decision making, or rigidity and unyielding diktat at the other, are compatible with what is best for patients.

Clinical guidelines are one of the basic tools for clinical decision making and for quality assurance in clinical practice. They will become important, therefore, in clinical governance and local medical regulation. This book, written by experts, tells working clinicians all they need to know about guidelines. It should be reassuring and practically helpful, it is certainly most timely.

Sir Donald Irvine CBE
February 1999

Preface

Clinicians have made use of guidelines in various forms since the days of Hippocrates, taking advice through learned texts and the recommendations of opinion leaders. More recently, and particularly over the past decade, clinical practice guidelines have taken on a different form from textbooks and reports from specialist and professional associations. Initially as consensus statements, but more recently as explicit statements of evidence linked to recommendations for practice, guidelines have become a separate entity, seeming to gain in importance as professionals face the challenge of improving quality of care and demonstrating that improvement is occurring.

It is this combination of challenges that led us to bring this collection of edited chapters together. The increase in the number and range of clinical guidelines has not been without its critics. Some health professionals regard guidelines as a threat, fearing if they do not comply with them they will be at risk of litigation. This is not a concern to be ignored and others have considered the matter in great detail.[1]

But many other concerns relate to the perceived loss of options for variations in clinical practice to take account of the health professional's and patient's circumstances and wishes. The use of guidelines clearly has implications for the methods used by health professionals to share information with patients and assist them in making decisions about their care. Furthermore, there are concerns about the number and quality of guidelines available, and the frequent failure of efforts to implement guideline recommendations.

Therefore, the purpose of this book is to share knowledge and best practice on the development, dissemination and implementation of clinical practice guidelines, drawing on examples from primary and secondary care including both local and national projects. The book is also offered as a resource for those who are responsible for guideline development and implementation. But more especially it is for those in

[1] Hurwitz B (1998) *Clinical Guidelines and the Law: negligence, discretion and judgment.* Radcliffe Medical Press, Oxford.

clinical practice in medicine, nursing and the professions allied to medicine, whose task it is to take evidence into practice for individual patient care.

Allen Hutchinson
Richard Baker
February 1999

List of contributors

Professor Allen Hutchinson, Professor of Public Health, ScHARR, University of Sheffield

Dr Richard Baker, Director, Eli Lilley Audit Centre, Department of General Practice, University of Leicester

Dr Gene Feder, Senior Lecturer in General Practice, Queen Mary and Westfield College, University of London

Dr Alan Breen, Director of Research, Anglo-European College of Chiropractice, Bournemouth

Professor Martin Eccles, Professor of Clinical Effectiveness, Centre for Health Services Research, University of Newcastle

Dr Bernard Higgins, Consultant Chest Physician, Freeman Hospital, Newcastle-Upon-Tyne

Dr Philip Adams, Consultant Cardiologist, Royal Victoria Infirmary, Newcastle-Upon-Tyne

Professor David Thompson, Professor of Nursing, Department of Health Studies, University of York

Professor Alison Kitson, Director, National Institute for Nursing and Centre for Practice and Development Research, Radcliffe Infirmary, Oxford

Aileen McIntosh, Research Fellow, Section of Public Health, ScHARR, University of Sheffield

François Cluzeau, Lecturer, Health Care Evaluation Unit, St George's Hospital Medical School, University of London

Professor Peter Littlejohns, Director, Health Care Evaluation Unit, St George's Hospital Medical School, University of London

Professor Ian Watt, Dissemination Manager, NHS Centre for Reviews and Dissemination, University of York

Dr Vicki Entwistle, Senior Research Fellow, Health Services Research Unit, University of Aberdeen

Dr Amanda Sowden, Senior Research Fellow, NHS Centre for Reviews and Dissemination, University of York

Elaine Taylor-Whilde, Chief Executive, Association for Quality in Health Care, Aldermaston

Dr Nicholas Hicks, Consultant in Public Health Medicine, Oxfordshire Health Authority, Honorary Senior Clinical Lecturer, Oxford University

Dr Francine Cheater, Senior Lecturer, Eli Lilley Audit Centre, Department of General Practice, University of Leicester

Acknowledgements

We would like to thank all of our colleagues who gave their time in contributions to this book, particularly for their unstinting attention to the editor's comments.

Many staff of Sheffield University School of Health and Related Research provided help and advice and we thank them for their assistance. Catherine Grinold bore the brunt of the editing process with great fortitude and we are most grateful to her for her support.

1
What are clinical practice guidelines?

Allen Hutchinson and Richard Baker

Improving and ensuring the quality of care is an important tenet of clinical practice, although quality improvement is often a complex process which requires considerable support and encouragement. One important starting point for improving quality is the provision of evidence and guidance on the effectiveness of treatments and care management, in ways which health professionals find clear and easy to use. An increasingly popular approach is the production of clinical practice guidelines.

The purpose of this book is to take a practical look at the development and implementation of guidelines. It is oriented towards doctors, nurses, allied health professions, and those who support them managerially. The contributing authors adopt a critical perspective, considering the weaknesses as well as the strengths of guidelines and make suggestions for improving the process where appropriate. While naturally focused on British clinical practice, drawing on the experience of a number of projects in the UK to examine the value of guidelines, there is much reference to international work on guideline development and implementation, and many of the lessons are appropriate in any developed health service.

Introduction

An increasing number of guidelines are being published nationally and internationally. In the English language alone the numbers run into thousands, with many duplications and with variations in quality that concern users and developers alike. This introductory chapter will take a practical overview of the concepts, values, uses and limitations of guidelines, beginning with the questions – what are guidelines and why might they be useful?

A dictionary definition of the word guideline is *'an indication of course that should be followed'*.[1] Authoritative statements or recommendations about the course to be followed by the health professional are not new. The aphorisms of the Hippocratic school are an early variety of guidelines, giving such advice as the following:

> It is unwise to prophesy either death or recovery in acute diseases.

and

> In acute diseases employ drugs very seldom and only at the beginning.[2]

The authority of statements of this type rested on the standing and respect accorded to the author, and they have been the bedrock of professional practice for generations. They remain, of course, the currency of clinical textbooks, for example:

> Physiotherapy (in the management of emphysema) may be helpful during exacerbations associated with bronchial infection to encourage expectoration. Regular exercise should be encouraged to increase mobility.[3]

So it can be argued that guidelines have been part of clinical practice for many generations, and can be found in the statements of professional associations and colleges throughout the world, in addition to textbooks and the advice of the great clinical teachers. But in recent years the concept of what guidelines are and what they are intended for has changed quite radically.

In any modern definition of clinical practice guidelines the common themes are:

- a systematic approach
- support for clinical decision making
- concern with specific clinical problems.

A useful starting point in considering the question 'what are guidelines?' is the often quoted definition of the Institute of Medicine, which first appeared in a report on guidelines[4] published in the US at a time when they were becoming widely available (although less so in other western healthcare services). Clinical practice guidelines were defined in that report as:

systematically developed statements to assist practitioner and patient decisions about appropriate healthcare for specific clinical circumstances.

This definition highlights the principle that clinical practice guidelines exist to provide guidance in such a way as to *assist* practitioners – clinicians of all types, including nurses, allied health professions and doctors – so that they can make decisions with and for patients who have identified and important clinical problems.

The other key element of the definition is that guideline statements are systematically developed. Suddenly, authority is not enough, but a particular process must be followed if a statement is to be classed as a guideline. Importantly, also, the definition makes it clear that guidelines are also important in decision making by patients as well as by clinicians.

Much of this book will be concerned with the practical details of this process and how the resulting statements and recommendations can be used by practitioners and patients. It is not intended to provide a 'how to do it guide', since there is no one perfect solution to this complex area. Rather, a practical application of theory is presented through examples of work undertaken within the National Health Service (NHS), supported by evidence on the development and implementation of guidelines.

But why this apparently sudden change of emphasis and the need for new definitions?

Why might guidelines be useful?

There are four principal reasons for the increased interest in the development and use of guidelines:

1 shared clinical decision making and increasing teamwork

2 the expanding evidence base of clinical practice

3 the information technology revolution

4 inappropriate variation in clinical practice.

Shared decision making

Of the reasons for the increased interest in guidelines, the first, and perhaps most fundamental, is the recognition that clinical decisions should be open, shared with patients and with other colleagues participating in care. Few clinicians work in isolation any more. Even in a rural general practice or a small community hospital, the doctor, nurse or physiotherapist will be providing care that links with the care of other professionals as part of a comprehensive package. Such sequences of care are sometimes described as 'care pathways', and embody an approach that requires all who are providing care to be aware of each other's roles in order to provide consistent care and advice. Some means of sharing that agreed, up-to-date care has to be found and one is to use a clinical practice guideline, which can guide the direction of care across professional boundaries.

In the past, health professionals have tended to make decisions for the patient, rather than with the patient. This has applied particularly in the area of diagnostics, but also more generally in the field of treatment. As interest in shared decision making has become more common, there has been an increasing need for explicit guidance which can be shared with individual patients. Guidelines in a suitable format may be able to meet the needs of patients for information to support their decision making. If more widely disseminated they may also contribute to increasing the knowledge of people not receiving healthcare. Public response to the publication by the Royal College of General Practitioners of clinical guidelines on the management of acute low back pain[5] demonstrated the considerable level of interest in knowing more about the subject, with the principal recommendations appearing in many popular publications, including those in minority languages. In the extensive programme of guideline development supported by the Agency for Health Care Policy and Research (AHCPR) in the US in recent years, a patient version of the guideline was routinely produced. For example, in the guideline entitled *Depression is a Treatable Illness*,[6] evidence-based guidance was given to patients that:

Antidepressant medicines are not addictive or habit forming. They work in severe depression and may be useful in mild to moderate depression.

Nevertheless, although at first sight the sharing of decisions with patients may appear a natural and beneficial step, there are arguments that indicate a need for caution. Different patients may want different amounts of information, and health professionals can find it difficult to present complex details in forms that can be easily understood.[7]

The expanding evidence base of clinical practice

In addition to facilitating shared decision making between patient and health professional, guidelines may also have a role in facilitating the sharing of decisions between groups of professionals caring for the same patient. The enormous expansion in available evidence about what constitutes good practice has been one of the remarkable features of healthcare in the past decade. It has been estimated that approximately two million articles are now published each year in the international clinical press, and the number of new journals is increasing. Indeed, in response to this information overload a new type of journal has emerged that summarises and reviews work published in other journals, a clear indication that it is becoming impossible to keep informed of relevant literature in any particular field by relying on original studies in journals. For the generalist the challenge is even greater, for it is just not possible to keep abreast of the range of new results arising from clinical research across the world for a wide range of clinical topics.

Not only is it difficult to keep up to date with new findings but it has become increasingly clear that the quality of many studies is inadequate to permit the practitioner to rely on single studies as guides to clinical practice. Without some form of systematic review and interpretation of the findings, presented in an accessible form, it is possible for the practitioner to believe that a form of treatment evaluated in a research study is effective, when in reality it is at best ineffective and perhaps even dangerous. The international movement to assess evidence through the rapidly expanding Cochrane Collaboration is an increasingly effective response to this problem. But for the busy, practising clinician it has also become clear that evidence requires interpretation if it is to be put to good use in specific clinical circumstances. Evidence of effectiveness of an intervention in one clinical subgroup may not always be directly transferable to another. Clinical guidelines are one means of presenting research findings to the clinician in an accessible manner following interpretation of the available evidence.

The information technology revolution

Information technology has played an exiting part in bringing evidence on effective healthcare to the attention of clinicians and patients. It is now possible to access information on the management of a wide range of clinical subjects. The AHCPR makes much of its documentation available on the World Wide Web and it is accessible to clinicians and patients alike (*http://www.ahcpr.gov/*). Many UK professional associations and colleges are following suit, and the European Union has put substantial resources into supporting the information technology research required to enable guidelines to be routinely available on screen.

An increasing number of patients and patient organisations have easy access to this material through information technology developments such as the World Wide Web. In some clinical disciplines, it is not uncommon for the practitioner to consult with a patient who is well briefed on the latest evidence about treatments.

Inappropriate variation in clinical practice

The fourth reason for increased interest in the development and use of clinical guidelines is perhaps the most uncomfortable, for clinicians and the general public alike. There is ample evidence that there are substantial variations in the process of care in most fields of clinical practice, some of which lead to significant adverse effects on the health of patients. Of course, by no means all variation in clinical practice is inappropriate. For example, in many aspects of care, evidence is not yet available to determine which intervention is the most effective in a specific clinical situation, a problem of concern to a number of contributing authors, for example in Chapters 2, 4 and 5.

It must also be recognised that patients differ both in the details of their conditions and in their psychological responses to illness and their preferences for alternative treatments. Furthermore, a substantial number of patients will have more than one condition, and in these circumstances there may be very good reasons for taking a clinical approach that does not follow guidance offered by a condition-specific guideline. Variation in clinical practice is therefore appropriate in many circumstances.

However, evidence from small area variations and the clinical audits in which most health professionals have participated in recent years have identified variation in clinical practice as a significant problem in the provision of healthcare, with evidence of inexplicable variation in practice still present when factors such as case mix and socio-demographic characteristics have been taken into account. It is increasingly clear that for some patients it is the place where they live that determines the type of care they receive. Even when resources are adequate there is still variation which may be inappropriate. Guidelines, if properly implemented, may make the effective management of clinical care increasingly possible by reducing inappropriate variation and improving efficiency (a role in which managers have a legitimate interest although it is often cast as cost containment).

Thus, guidelines are seen by an increasing number of clinicians and professional groups as a means of making evidence and evidence-based recommendations easily available to the busy nurse, doctor, physiotherapist and other colleagues. They are an important component of the overall quality improvement steps which professional associations and Royal Colleges are taking to maintain the standard of clinical practice. They will also have an important role within the clinical governance of healthcare organisations. Therefore, a combination of powerful forces is making the greater availability of guidelines inevitable, and it follows that practitioners need to understand how they are developed and used, and the implications.

Tools not rules

One of the most acute concerns of clinicians, especially doctors, is that guideline use will suffocate new ideas or experimental developments in treatment. The phrase 'tools not rules' was coined by an American group of clinicians to illustrate how guidelines can sit comfortably with the need for decision making for individual patients, a process which inevitably requires an interpretation of recommendations that reflect the individual patient's circumstances. This element of joint decision making is an essential part of interpreting recommendations, and Cheater and Baker explore many of these issues in detail in Chapter 11.

Guidelines are therefore intended as tools to assist,[4] rather than replace, decision making. They are available both to support the management of the individual patient and to be taken account of in the development of local health services by bringing up to date, evaluated evidence and recommendations together in an accessible form. By making these links to evidence, guidelines can sometimes make strong statements about what should not be done under particular circumstances (for instance, the use of a particular antibiotic for a patient in a particular age group). More usually the recommendations will make proposals which should be considered as front line management in uncomplicated cases, taking into account the strength of the evidence. For example, in the Scottish Intercollegiate Guidelines Network (SIGN) guideline on the care of patients with chronic leg ulcer,[8] clinicians are advised as shown in Box 1.1.

Box 1.1: The SIGN guideline on care of chronic leg ulcer

'Pooling the results of studies of multilayer compression compared to single layer compression demonstrates an increase in complete healing when a multilayer high compression system is used'.

thus

'multilayer bandaging is recommended'.

But also that 'there is good evidence that the type of dressing has no effect on ulcer healing'.

thus

'Simple adherent dressings are recommended in the treatment of venous ulcers as no specific dressing has been shown to improve healing rates'.

Guidelines also have a place in the management of complicated cases but clinical interpretation of the specific circumstances is paramount. Such dilemmas abound in clinical practice. For instance, in an older man with congestive cardiac failure, asthma and a chronic leg ulcer, decisions may have to be made which balance the recommendations for each of the problems and priorities for treatment, perhaps leading to decisions on management which do not match one or more of the relevant guidelines. Similar circumstances might apply when front line treatments fail and there is a need for an innovative approach in an unusual case. Thus, the view that guidelines are 'tools not rules'.

These arguments are also a riposte to the criticism (usually from doctors) that guidelines are a form of 'cookbook medicine'. On the contrary, it is increasingly obvious that the interpretation of population data in the application of evidence and recommendations to the case of an individual patient requires enhanced clinical and scientific skills, not less. We return to these important issues in our concluding Chapter 12 where we consider how guidelines may influence future everyday practice.

What makes a good guideline?

There are several sets of criteria for judging the value and usefulness of a clinical guideline. These relate to:

- choice of subject
- the methodology used to bring the evidence together and to make recommendations
- the professional process by which the guideline was developed and disseminated.

Choosing the subject

In the UK, it has been recognised that national guidelines should only be produced for a limited number of important topics[9] (developed, say, by one or more of the Royal Colleges or professional associations). The choice of subjects should be guided by five principles:

1 where there is considerable morbidity, disability or mortality

2 where treatment offers good potential for reduction in morbidity, disability or mortality

3 where there is wide variation in clinical practice across the country

4 where services are resource intensive: either high cost/low volume, high cost/high volume, or low cost/high volume

5 where there are significant boundary issues between services or professions.

To these might be added:

- the potential for reaching consensus, and
- the potential for effective implementation.

For the purposes of both national and local guideline development it is important to have a set of decision criteria such as these in order to make efficient use of resources, not least because much valuable professional time can be spent (and wasted) on guideline development. Moreover, as a number of contributing authors convincingly demonstrate, even more time may be spent on implementation if guidelines are to improve patient care. So, not only must guideline development be prioritised in terms of the relative importance of the topic but serious consideration must be given to usability of the product, otherwise it will, at best, languish on a bookshelf.

Development methods

New methods of evaluating evidence, linked with the information technology revolution and creation of centres for evidence evaluation such as the Cochrane Collaboration and the UK Centre for Reviews and Dissemination, now provide the opportunity to access research evidence which has been graded for quality and reliability. This has enabled guideline developers to present a synthesis of the international evidence on a particular subject and link it to the recommendation in a way which is unambiguous to the reader. Using the national guideline on acute back pain as a model for this approach, Breen and Feder demonstrate in Chapter 2 how evidence is accessed and interpreted.

It is only relatively recently that clinical practice guideline developers have begun to be explicit about production methods and incorporated explicit links between evidence and guideline recommendations.[10] Eccles and his colleagues have been responsible for refining methods of the guideline development process in Britain by rigorously evaluating evidence, and by paying particular attention to group process and transparency in determining recommendations from evidence. They explain their methods in Chapter 3 using experience of developing guidelines for recurrent wheeze (asthma) and for recurrent chest pain (angina of effort).

Although guidelines as expressions of good professional practice have been available for many years, they tended to be created by opinion formers, without explicit reference to the evidence base on which recommendations were founded. A group of specialists in a field would come together to share their wisdom and publish it for the benefit of the 'less wise'. This approach is no longer regarded as adequate, not least because there is some reason to suspect that the most up-to-date evidence is not always incorporated into such discussions and therefore validity may be poor.[11]

From the perspective of the developer, in Chapter 4, Thompson and Kitson demonstrate some of the practical difficulties encountered in trying to provide guidance when the evidence base is weak, and demonstrate how survey methods can support the process of deriving consensus recommendations. By contrast, in her exploration of consensus methods in Chapter 5, McIntosh examines the strengths and weaknesses of the consensus approach to guidelines development, and identifies means by which the approach can be strengthened.

Who produces guidelines?

It has been suggested that over 20 000 clinical guidelines of varying type have been produced in recent years in North America. There may be almost as many available to clinicians in the European Union, with its similar population size. The Dutch College of General Practitioners, for example, has produced almost 70 guidelines since its first guideline on the management of diabetes was published in 1989. Certainly in the UK, there is increasing development activity among the Royal Colleges, the professional societies and associations and research teams. Add to this the activity which is driven locally by the NHS through health authorities and health boards, hospitals and local quality and clinical audit groups, and the scale of the activity looks daunting.

As Cluzeau and Littlejohns point out in their international work for the assessment of the quality of guidelines in Chapter 6, local production resulted in many guidelines being produced for very similar purposes, often of rather indifferent quality with only tenuous links between evidence and recommendations.

This is not always the case – for instance the first guidelines of the North of England Evidence Based Guideline Development Project were commissioned by the local regional health authority. The debate over who develops which type of guideline is not yet settled although increasingly health policy is dictating that national guidelines will be used as the basis for local development. In Scotland, guidelines are developed jointly by SIGN under the banner of 'national clinical guideline(s)' while in England and Wales these will be the domain of the National Institute for Clinical Excellence (NICE).[12]

Yet there may still be a place for developing evidence-based guidelines at a local level, despite the doubt that local groups have the resources to support such development. Perhaps the local role is one of placing national guidelines in a local context, a task which might also incorporate decisions on access that will vary according to the availability of resources but will still be guided by the evidence on appropriate clinical practice. Hutchinson and Feder examine the arguments and the methods for taking this approach in Chapter 7.

Improving patient care

Since the prime purpose of clinical guidelines is to contribute to improvements in patient care, the method of implementing guidelines is an important factor in any discussion on the subject. But experience with clinical behaviour change has repeatedly shown that it is difficult for health professionals to alter their practice, even when they are aware of new evidence which supports change in a particular direction.[13] This recognition has spawned considerable international research on best use of available resources.

In Chapter 8, Watt, Entwistle and Sowden review the international evidence on what we know about the best means of taking evidence into practice. There are still many unknowns although the considerable increase in research activity should begin to provide some answers in the near future. Nevertheless, there is already enough knowledge to begin to direct implementation activity and Chapters 8, 9 and 10 all use an evidence-based approach towards taking evidence into practice.

At the local level (where implementation is what matters) the place for developing evidence-based clinical guidelines is also considered by Taylor-Whilde and Hutchinson (Chapter 9) as they report on a local process for implementation which draws together national and local guidelines, together with innovative methods on behaviour change arising from the management research literature.

Many health services and systems are now exploring methods of taking evidence into practice through some form of contracting or commissioning of healthcare. From primary care groups in England and Wales to health maintenance organisations in the United States, commissioning methods are being used which use evidence-based practice as their starting point while trying to ensure value-for-money. These methods are in early stages in the UK, but Hicks demonstrates in Chapter 10 that it is possible to commission evidence-based healthcare, given the right resources and skills.

Implementation, however, eventually comes down to the interaction between patient and clinician or clinical team. The patient perspective, examined by Cheater and Baker in Chapter 11, is followed by our analysis of the opportunities and the acknowledged difficulties of using guidelines in everyday clinical practice. This book takes up the challenge of trying to make both sense and use of this expanding field of clinical practice.

References

1   Macdonald AM (ed) (1972) *Chambers Twentieth Century Dictionary.* Chambers, Edinburgh.
2   Lloyd GER (1978) *Hippocratic Writings.* Penguin, Harmondsworth.

3 Edwards CRW *et al.* (eds) (1995) *Davidson's Principles and Practice of Medicine*. Churchill Livingstone, Edinburgh.

4 Field MJ and Lohr KN (eds) (1992) *Guidelines for Clinical Practice: From Development to Use*. Institute of Medicine/National Academy Press, Washington DC.

5 Waddell G, Feder G and Lewis M (1997) Systematic reviews of bed rest and advice to stay active for acute low back pain. *British Journal of General Practice*, **47**: 647–52.

6 Agency for Health Care Policy and Research (1993) *Depression is a Treatable Illness. A Patient's Guide*. AHCPR/US Department of Health and Human Services, Rockville, MD.

7 Baker R and Feder G (1997) Clinical guidelines: where next? *International Journal for Quality in Health Care*, **9**: 399–404.

8 Scottish Intercollegiate Guidelines Network (1998) *The Care of Patients with Chronic Leg Ulcer*. SIGN, Edinburgh.

9 National Health Service Executive (1996) *Clinical Guidelines: Using Clinical Guidelines to Improve Patient Care within the NHS*. NHS Executive, Leeds.

10 Woolf S, DiGuiseppi CG, Atkins D and Kamerow DB (1996) Developing evidence-based clinical practice guidelines: lessons learned by the US Preventive Services Task Force. *Annual Review of Public Health*, **17**: 511–38.

11 Grimshaw J and Russell IT (1993) Effect of clinical guidelines on medical practice: a systematic review of rigorous evaluations. *Lancet*, **342**: 1317–22.

12 Secretary of State for Health (1998) *A First Class Service: quality in the new NHS*. The Stationery Office, London.

13 Oxman AD, Thomson MA and Davis DA (1995) No magic bullets: a systematic review of 102 trials of interventions to improve professional practice. *Canadian Medical Association Journal*, **153**: 1423–31.

2
Where does the evidence come from?

Alan Breen and Gene Feder

Since more than two million clinical research articles are published annually worldwide, accessing and evaluating evidence for guidelines is a complicated task. Here, the authors look at some of the principles and practicalities of finding relevant evidence and offer some straightforward guidance. By using the experience gained from the English acute low back pain guideline, Breen and Feder also provide a pragmatic model for guideline developers who have only limited resources and wish to use available evidence sources as a means of making rapid progress.

Introduction

Clinical guidelines are not new. Clinicians have made recommendations about good practice to other clinicians for millennia but particular recent developments are the systematic collection of scientific evidence of effective practice and the formulation of guidelines explicitly based on that evidence. Although much of clinical practice suffers from lack of rigorous research, it is distressing that even the recent history of medical practice is littered with examples of well-researched treatments that are not applied to patient care.[1] Guidelines that link recommendations to research are one tool for bringing evidence of effective practice to the attention of clinicians; they can also make explicit the uncertainty underlying particular diagnosis and treatment decisions.[2]

The main aim of this chapter is to describe a process for collecting and evaluating clinical research evidence for the formulation of guideline recommendations. The process includes characterising the main clinical decisions which the guidelines will address, setting criteria for inclusion of evidence, systematically searching for relevant studies, summarising their conclusions, and deriving recommendations. This model has evolved from the discipline of clinical epidemiology[3] and has been used in North America[2] and, more recently, in UK guidelines.[4] We have drawn extensively on our own experience of developing national guidelines for the primary care management of acute back pain.[5]

Shifting the balance between consensus and evidence

The growing availability of well-designed clinical trials increases the potential for guideline recommendations to be based on evidence, moving beyond a simple consensus of experts in the field. Sole reliance on expert knowledge and interpretation of all relevant trials is risky as is demonstrated by the lag before robust research evidence is usually incorporated into expert recommendations. For example, thrombolyis for acute myocardial infarction was not recommended in editorials and textbooks until several years after the studies reporting its effectiveness had been published.

The validity of a guideline does not depend on the clinical, or even the research, expertise of the development group, but on a reproducible, relatively unbiased method of identifying and assessing the relevant evidence, and explicit linkage of recommendations to the underlying evidence. The development of evidence-linked guidelines does not eliminate the need for consensus, as the development group and external referees essentially have to reach a consensus on specific recommendations. But the development of evidence-linked guidelines where the evidence is explicitly linked to each recommendation means that the interpretation of research evidence is more transparent and more open to challenge.

Key clinical decisions

Guidelines are tools for clinical decision making. Before collecting evidence for recommendations, guideline developers need to characterise not only the clinical area that they want to address, but also the specific decisions on which they want to make recommendations and bring to bear the relevant evidence. Focusing the guideline on specific decisions will prevent collection of research evidence that may be interesting, but not patient- or treatment-centred. For example, debates about aetiology outside the context of specific prevention or treatment decisions would be best left to textbooks or review articles. Identifying decisions for guideline development is analogous to the formulation of 'well-built clinical questions' which underpin effective evidence searches to support individual clinical decisions.[6]

In the case of the recently developed UK acute back pain guidelines, the key decisions were: which diagnostic methods and when to use them in primary care, how to 'triage' patients presenting with acute back pain, and appropriate treatments in the first six weeks. These were broken down into more detailed questions (e.g. should bedrest be recommended? what analgesics are effective?) that guided the search for evidence.

Finding the evidence

Bibliographic databases allow us to identify an ever growing proportion of relevant diagnostic and treatment studies in specific clinical areas. Developing an effective search strategy is a skill which improves with experience and, if you are relatively new to database searching, support of a medical librarian in refining the search strategy will save time. Search terms, languages of papers, review period, and types of studies should be decided prior to carrying out the search. The selection of studies to be included in the review is made according to criteria set out in advance, depending on what type of clinical decision is being addressed. For example, evidence about diagnostic tests comes from cross-sectional studies, whereas treatment decisions are most firmly based on randomised controlled trials. If there is a shortage of the types of studies that provide the best evidence, then other types may be included. In the case of treatment decisions, case control or other quasi-experimental studies may have to be considered.

A search of MEDLINE and EMBASE over a specific time period (depending on resources available) will identify a variable proportion of studies published in peer-reviewed journals. Subsequent citation-tracking of the titles selected using the Science Citation index will identify other publications which may provide additional evidence. This may prompt a revision of search terms and a second MEDLINE search. The reference base obtained can then be compared with the personal bibliographies of available experts and checked against a hand search of the references offered in (at least) the main articles found. Identification of unpublished studies by correspondence with experts in the field helps counterbalance publication bias which favours trials with positive results. Finally, this can be followed by a second hand search of the references thrown up. For specialist areas, there may be other bibliographic databases suggested by members of the guideline development group.

Exhaustive searches of this kind are required to support an authoritative guideline, but the resources for the search and appraisal of the evidence are only a realistic prospect for national, or high quality regional guidelines, such as the North of England angina guidelines that were based on rigorous searching and appraisal of studies from one bibliographic database (MEDLINE) (*see* Chapter 3). Central to this stage of guidelines development is the construction of a 'rolling bibliography' from which, through elimination of studies which do not meet pre-set quality criteria, a definitive evidence base evolves.

When evidence-based guidelines are already available on a clinical topic, resources are better spent adapting and updating the guidelines rather than *de novo* development. Systematic searches are still necessary for new studies. If there is new evidence the development group can then review recommendations.

Appraising the evidence

Once published research relevant to the guidelines has been identified, the studies need to be appraised for soundness or validity. This appraisal process becomes more formidable with an increasing number of studies, and more complex if a range of research methodologies is included in the evidence base for the guidelines: randomised controlled trials, case control studies, cohort studies. As randomised controlled trials (RCTs) are the least biased method for comparing the effectiveness of treatments, *treatment* recommendations should be based on these trials if good quality studies are available. The grading of research studies by methodology (*see* Box 2.1) reflects the greater weight given to RCTs. Yet, even if RCTs are available, they may not include categories of patients, such as the elderly,[7] for whom the guidelines may be intended, or they may not provide information about long-term outcomes. Therefore, large cohort studies tracking the impact of risk factors (e.g. Framingham data on cardiovascular risk) or case control studies (e.g. linking the prescribing of non-steroidal anti-inflammatory drugs and the prescribing of antihypertensive therapy[8] may be helpful in complementing the results of RCTs. The grading of studies by methodology is not the same as appraising the *quality* of those studies which are identified as appropriate for formulation of recommendations and either excluding or giving less weight to studies that are poorly designed.

Box 2.1: Features used to assess quality of trial reports

A Validated scale (higher = better)

Feature	*Points*
RANDOMISATION	
• randomised	+1
• method described and appropriate	+1
• inappropriate method	−1
DOUBLE-BLINDING	
• double blind	+1
• masking described and appropriate	+1
• inappropriate method	−1
DROPOUTS AND WITHDRAWALS	
• numbers and reasons for withdrawal	+1

B Individual components known to affect estimates of intervention efficacy

Generation of random numbers
Adequate if generated by computer, random numbers table, shuffled cards or tossed coins and minimisation

Concealment of treatment allocation
Allocation to intervention or control concealed from investigators up to the point of treatment

---

Weighted quality criteria have been developed for appraisal of different types of clinical research studies, although they are not applicable uniformly or consistently. There is no universal grading system for the quality of treatment trials – appraisal of trial quality is important because of the likelihood of bias in poor quality trials. A recent study of the quality of randomised trials, using a validated scale (*see* Box 2.1) showed that poor quality trials were associated with increased estimates of treatment benefit.[9] Decisions about minimal quality standards for studies to be included in the evidence base require consensus on the part of the development group, and these decisions will be driven partly by overall availability of relevant studies. The development group needs to decide whether they have the resources or competence to undertake new systematic reviews. From the perspective of guidelines developers, the increasing number of published systematic reviews and the promise by the Cochrane Collaboration of high quality continuously updated reviews is a great relief. They offer guideline developers an alternative to undertaking the reviews themselves. Good systematic reviews are based on time-consuming and rigorous search and appraisal methods. When data from different trials are comparable, quantitative summaries (meta-analyses) of diagnostic or treatment effects are possible. Finding systematic reviews has become easier because of coding on bibliographic databases and the development of World Wide Web sites by groups like the Cochrane Collaboration. If guideline developers are to use systematic reviews, they need to be appraised for validity and appropriateness just as much as do primary research studies (e.g. the Dutch criteria for systematic reviews) (*see* Box 2.2).

Box 2.2: Sources of systematic reviews on the Internet

The Cochrane Library
A collection of databases of the *Cochrane Database of Systematic Reviews* and critical commentaries on selected reviews.
http://www.medlib.co

Effective Health Care Bulletins
Summaries of systematic reviews produced by the NHS Centre for Reviews and Dissemination.
http://www.york.ac.uk/inst/crd

Clinical Guidelines from the US Agency for Health Care Policy and Research
Full text guidelines which include summaries of systematic reviews on which they are based. The AHCPR is no longer producing guidelines, but will produce evidence reports on which guidelines can be based.
http//text.nlm.nih.gov

Netting the evidence
Maintained by the School of Health and Related Research (ScHARR) in Sheffield – this site links to many reviewed/refereed sources of evidence.
http://www.shef.ac.uk/~scharr/ir/netting.html

From evidence to recommendation

The identification and appraisal of evidence on which to base guideline recommendations is a largely technical task. Their satisfactory achievement depends on methodological competence and sufficient resources. The formulation of recommendations is intrinsically more controversial, since this entails the interpretation of evidence and making decisions about clinical policy. Below, we take a recent national guideline development project as a case study, exemplifying the challenge of formulating recommendations and also casting some light on the politics of guideline development (e.g. *see* Chapter 3).

National acute back pain guidelines development: a case study

Background

The development of the acute low back pain guidelines in England was a collaboration between the Royal College of General Practitioners, Chartered Society of Physiotherapists, British Osteopathic and Chiropractors, together with an important contribution from orthopaedic surgery and a patient's organisation. It is an example of how controversy can largely be resolved after the evaluation of a large heterogeneous evidence base.

In 1992, the Department of Health, recognising the unsatisfactory nature of services for sufferers of low back pain, commissioned the Clinical Standards Advisory Group (CSAG) to investigate and make recommendations about standards of care for the condition. Central to the CSAG brief was the issue of access to and availability of services that could be provided by the NHS.[10] Although the CSAG back pain group's remit was not to develop guidelines, its evidence review, much of it previously considered by the Agency for Health Care Policy Research in the United States (AHCPR),[11] led it to make recommendations about the clinical management of low back pain management which were inextricably linked to service and resource issues.

By the time the CSAG report was published there was growing recognition that recommendations about clinical management should be explicitly linked to underlying evidence,[12] but despite using the AHCPR evidence base, the CSAG back pain group did not make such explicit links. Furthermore, new trials of low back pain management added to the case for producing evidence-linked guidelines.

The Royal College of General Practitioners (RCGP), in collaboration with professional bodies representing the major professional groups managing back pain in primary care, undertook to update and address the evidence in the context of clinical practice guidelines separate from the service provision issues which had preoccupied the CSAG group. The focus of the guidelines was supporting individual clinical decisions. The objectives of the development group were:

- to provide evidence-based recommendations on the management of low back pain to the range of clinicians involved in first contact care

- to ensure a multidisciplinary approach to back pain management through the development and review process and through local implementation.

By inviting other professional groups with expertise in back pain management to join the development group (physiotherapists, chiropractors, osteopaths), the benefits of a rigorous evidence review were combined with the widest professional consensus yet seen in the production of national clinical guidelines, increasing their likelihood of multiprofessional acceptance.[5]

The development group started from the extensive AHCPR review which underpinned the American evidence-based guidelines (*see* Box 2.3) and undertook systematic reviews of further evidence published from January 1993 to April 1996 using standard search techniques and review methods. Additional material, including work in press, was obtained from a number of sources, particularly non-UK members of the Cochrane Collaboration on back pain and from other local UK guidelines.

Focused reviews

The development group made a pragmatic decision to repeat and/or update systematic reviews of four key treatment options for the patient presenting with acute simple back pain where there was still controversy about effectiveness and new evidence:

1 bedrest (complete review)

2 advice on staying active (complete review)

3 manipulation (update of AHCPR review)

4 exercise (update of AHCPR review).

Box 2.3: Criteria for quality appraisal of systematic reviews (details for application of these criteria can be found in Assendelft *et al.*, 1995[12])

Study selection
- description of inclusion and exclusion criteria
- search strategy
- emphasis on randomised controlled trial

Methodological quality assessment
- assessment of validity of RCTs
- number of reviewers
- blinding of reviewer(s)
- agreement of reviewer(s)

Intervention
- description of intervention(s)
- description of control intervention(s)

Data presentation
- outcome presentation
- statistical pooling
- discussion of power of negative RCTs

Evaluation
- overall conclusion
- discussion of heterogeneity of RCTs and outcomes

We compared our reviews to other recent systematic reviews of bedrest, manipulation[13] and exercise.[14] The existence of the AHCPR's extensive and relatively recent evidence base covering acute back pain management allowed us to avoid searching and reappraising research on other treatment and diagnostic decisions, except for searches of bibliographic databases for systematic reviews that had been published since the AHCPR search. These reviews were appraised using methodological quality criteria and compared to the AHCPR evidence. Lastly, two recent 'mega' analyses of the whole range of back pain treatment options,[15,16] which were in press as we were completing our guidelines, were used to check our reviews for any important inconsistencies. Essentially, we made a pragmatic decision driven by time and resource constraints not to 'start from scratch', while recognising that we might miss new studies outside the four areas which we systematically reviewed.

Conflicting evidence

Even before the development group had to grapple with recommendations, we had to face conflicting evidence from systematic reviews. For example, the effectiveness of manipulation emerged from a meta-analysis by Shekelle[17,18] and from our own review[19] but was contested in Koes'[13] review. All the reviews were methodologically sound and included largely the same trials. They differed in their judgement of trial quality and, in particular, to what extent methodological weaknesses in trials invalidated the positive effect that manipulation had on acute back pain in the majority of trials. The development group had to discuss these issues in detail before being able to produce recommendations.

Another example of ambiguous, if not actually conflicting, evidence came around the issue of advice about activity for patients with acute back pain. From a consideration of the AHCPR evidence base it was clear that research on exercise advice and advice to return to normal activity had been conflated, and it was therefore difficult to make recommendations about either. This ambiguity needed resolution and drove us to undertake a complete review of trials which tested advice about early resumption of normal activity.

'Activity' is not a MeSH term, complicating the search strategy. The reviewers searched MEDLINE from 1964 to April 1996 and EMBASE from 1980 to April 1996 under the general headings of 'back pain' or 'low back pain', 'randomised controlled trial', 'controlled clinical trial'', 'acute' or 'primary care', 'usual care/management' and 'exercise'. This search was supplemented by a personal bibliography, and a citation search from all relevant papers found in the initial search. Eight trials including advice to stay active were identified, showing consistently positive results in terms of satisfaction, subsequent healthcare use, return to work and subsequent chronic disability, although not in terms of initial recovery and pain level.[20] These results allowed the development group to recommend advice to stay active as an effective 'treatment' for patients with acute back pain.

Grading the evidence

Evidence does not speak for itself. To produce an evidence-based clinical guideline it must be both graded and converted into recommendations.

Grading of evidence statements is necessary because the strength of the evidence is an important factor in the strength of recommendations even if recommendations are not themselves graded. If evidence statements are not graded, the user is not able to distinguish largely consensual recommendations where studies are not available (or are of an unacceptably poor quality) from recommendations based on good quality studies with consistent findings.

Grading of evidence statements in guidelines combines a judgement about quality of studies included in the evidence base and, particularly for diagnostic and treatment recommendations, the appropriateness of the methodology (*see* Chapter 3). There is no universal grading system for the quality of treatment trials. Most combine features relating to potential biases (*see* Box 2.1) with a judgement about sample size, characteristics of the intervention(s) and appropriateness of analysis. Systematic reviews themselves can be graded by quality (*see* Box 2.4) and in the course of developing the acute back pain guidelines we searched and appraised systematic reviews which had appeared since the development of the AHCPR guidelines, checking if their conclusions conflicted with the evidence base of those guidelines.

For some interventions, such as spinal manipulation, the large number of trials and systematic reviews (and the status of manipulation as a 'complementary' therapy within UK practice) required repeated returns to the evidence with debates about study quality and conclusions before we could formulate an acceptable evidence statement. Even at the level of evidence statements, before recommendations are formulated, interpretation and consensus play a part, particularly where the evidence from trials is contradictory or controversial.

The grading of evidence statements in guidelines should be readily understandable as their function is to alert the casual reader or busy clinician to the strength or weakness of specific statements. An early attempt by the Canadian Task Force,[21] for example, offered three grades depending on the quality and type of studies (*see* Box 2.4). This form of

---

Box 2.4: Canadian Task Force evidence gradings

Level of evidence	*Criteria*
I	Well-designed randomised controlled trials, meta-analyses or systematic reviews
II	Well-designed non-randomised prospective or retrospective controlled studies
III	Uncontrolled studies or consensus

grading, with subdivisions, has found acceptance in some UK guidelines (e.g. *see* Chapter 3) where RCTs, meta-analyses and systematic reviews were the most suitable forms of evidence. The American AHCPR guidelines graded evidence by a four-point system. There are no studies demonstrating the superiority of one grading system over another.

We adopted a three-point scale for the UK acute back pain guidelines (*see* Box 2.5). As some of the statements in the guidelines about assessment of the patient and natural history were appropriately based on cohort studies, the grading was adapted to accommodate that methodology. Randomised controlled trials are not the 'gold standard' for assessment and natural history as they are for questions of treatment efficacy.

Box 2.5: RCGP back pain evidence gradings

*** Generally consistent finding in a majority of multiple acceptable studies

** Either based on a single acceptable study, or a weak or inconsistent finding in some multiple acceptable studies

* Limited scientific evidence which does not meet all the criteria of acceptable studies

---

'Acceptable' studies of therapy

- Randomised controlled trial
- Acute (<3/12) or recurrent cases
- Relevant to primary care
- At least 10 patients in each group
- Patient centred outcome(s)

'Acceptable' studies of assessment and natural history

- Prospective cohort study
- Acute or recurrent cases
- Relevant to primary care
- At least 100 patients
- At least one year follow up

Evidence into recommendations

This chapter is about finding, appraising and formulating evidence for guidelines, using the English acute low back pain guidelines as an example. But the story of these guidelines is incomplete without saying how the development group formulated its recommendations from the evidence. This process had two stages. First, evidence-linked statements were produced for each of the areas of care (assessment, drug therapy, bedrest, advice on staying active, manipulation and back exercise). Second, small multiprofessional subgroups prepared the recommendations in clinically important areas. These were then discussed and agreed by informal consensus. The interpretation of the evidence for some clinical decisions was controversial and formulation of recommendations is always the most difficult step in guidelines development. Yet, without the rigorous searching and appraising of relevant research and the colossal work of the AHCPR reviewers which underpinned its acute back pain guidelines, it would have been even more difficult to agree on recommendations acceptable to all the relevant professional groups. A comprehensive, unbiased evidence base, linked to specific recommendations, is a prerequisite for good quality guidelines.

References

1 Antman EM, Lau J, Kupeinick B, Mostellar F and Chaimers TC (1992) A comparison of results of meta-analyses of randomised controlled trials and recommendations of experts. *JAMA*, **268**: 240–8.

2 Field MJ and Lohr KN (eds) (1992) *Guidelines for Clinical Practice: From Development to Use*. Institute of Medicine/National Academy Press, Washington DC.

3 Sackett DL, Haynes RB, Guyatt GH and Tugwell P (1991) *Clinical Epidemiology: A Basic Science for Clinical Medicine*. Boston: Little, Brown.

4 Eccles M, Clapp Z, Grimshaw J *et al.* (1996) Developing valid guidelines: methodological and procedural issues from the North of England Evidence Based Guideline Development Project. *Quality in Health Care*, **5**: 44–50.

5 Royal College of General Practitioners (1996) *Clinical Guidelines for the Management of Acute Low Back Pain: Clinical Guidelines and Evidence Review*. RCGP, London.

6 Richardson WS, Wilson MC, Nishikawa J and Hayward RSA (1995) The well built clinical question: a key to evidence-based decisions (editorial). *ACP Journal Club*, **123**: A12–13.

7 Bugea G, Kumar A and Banerjee AK (1997) Exclusion of elderly people from clinical research: a descriptive study of published reports. BMJ, **315**: 1059.

8 Gurwitz JH, Avorn J, Bohn R, Glynn RJ, Monane M and Mogun H (1994) Initiation of anti-hypertensive treatment during nonsteroidal anti-inflammatory drug therapy. *JAMA*, **272**: 781–6.

9 Moher D, Pham B, Jones A *et al.* (1998) Does quality of reports of randomised trials affect estimates of intervention efficacy reported in meta-analyses? *Lancet*, **352**: 609–13.

10 Clinical Standards Advisory Group (1994) *Back Pain*. HMSO, London.

11 Agency for Health Care Policy and Research (1994) *Management Guidelines for Acute Low Back Pain*. AHCPR/US Department of Health and Human Services, Rockville, MD.

12 Assendelft WJJ, Koes BW, Knipschild P *et al.* (1995) The relationship between methodological quality and conclusions in reviews of spinal manipulation. *JAMA*, **274**: 1942–8.

13 Koes BW, Assendelft WJJ, van der Heijden GJMG and Bouter LM (1996) Spinal manipulation and mobilisation for low back pain: an updated systematic review of randomised clinical trials (systematic review). *Spine*, **21**: 2860–73.

14 Faas A *et al.* (1996) Exercises; which ones are worth trying, for which patients and when? (systematic review). *Spine*, **21**: 2874–9.

15 Evans G and Richards S (1996) *Low Back Pain: An Evaluation of Therapeutic Interventions* (mega-analysis). Health Care Evaluation Unit/University of Bristol, Bristol.

16 van Tulder MW, Koes BW and Bouter LM (eds) (1996) *Low back pain in primary care: Effectiveness of diagnostic and therapeutic interventions.* Institute for Extramural Studies, Amsterdam.

17 Shekelle P (1995) *Spinal manipulation and mobilisation for low back pain.* Paper presented to the International Forum for Primary Care Research on Low Back Pain, Seattle.

18 Shekelle PG, Adams AH, Chassim MR *et al.* (1992) Spinal manipulation for back pain. *Ann Int Med*, **117**: 590–8.

19 Waddell G, Feder G, Mcintosh A, Lewis M and Hutchinson A (1996) *Low Back Pain Evidence Review*. Royal College of General Practitioners, London.

20 Waddell G, Feder G and Lewis M (1997) Systematic reviews of bedrest and advice to stay active for acute low back pain. *British Journal of General Practitioners*, **47**: 647–52.

21 Canadian Task Force (1979) Task force classification of study designs. *Canadian Medical Association Journal*, **121**: 1193–254.

3

Developing evidence-based guidelines: experiences from the North of England Evidence-Based Guideline Development Project

Martin Eccles, Bernard Higgins and Philip Adams

Guideline development methods have changed rapidly over recent years, from the products of expert committees and the consensus conference to the evidence-based guideline with a specific methodological approach which is reproducible and explicit. Relatively few guideline projects have been as methodologically rigorous as the North of England Guideline Project. The project team's approach has enabled a detailed account to be made of the challenges faced by guideline developers. It contains valuable guidance based on the experience of producing two guidelines recommended for use in the National Health Service.

Introduction

With an increasing interest in clinical guidelines within the UK has come an increasing awareness of the methodological issues involved in guideline development, although reports of these methods are limited.[1] This chapter describes the experiences and methodological issues addressed during the development of explicit, evidence-based guidelines for two common chronic conditions; stable angina and recurrent wheeze in adults,[8-12] predominantly cared for in primary care and important because of their associated morbidity and mortality.[13] The aim is to present our experiences and the methodological issues addressed during the development process, both for those who are or may be involved in guideline development, and for those who wish to know more about the practicalities involved.

Woolf has described three main methods of guideline development: informal consensus, formal consensus and evidence-linked guideline development.[2] In *informal consensus* development, the method used most frequently in the UK, the guideline panel has poorly defined, often implicit, criteria for decision making. *Formal consensus* development methods, used by many consensus development conferences and Delphi groups, provide 'greater structure to the analytical process' but still fail to provide 'an explicit linkage between recommendations and quality of evidence'.[2] *Evidence-linked* guideline development requires the explicit linkage of recommendations to the quality of the supporting evidence.[3,4] This allows the user to make an informed choice about whether to comply with individual recommendations within the guideline by taking account of the category of supporting evidence.

Guidelines are said to be valid if 'when followed they lead to the health gains and costs predicted for them'.[5] It has previously been argued that evidence-linked guideline development is one of three developmental prerequisites necessary to maximise guideline validity,[6] the other two being systematic review of the evidence and guideline development occurring within an appropriately multidisciplinary group. These methods are unlikely to be used at a local (as opposed to a regional or national) level as necessary skills are usually not available and local groups should therefore concentrate on identifying valid regional or national guidelines which they can then adapt to their local needs.[7] Unfortunately, such valid guidelines are few and descriptions of their development in the UK non-existent.

Setting up the guideline development project

To achieve successfully the task of guideline development it proved necessary to convene three groups:

1 a project team

2 a project management group

3 two guideline development groups.

The *project team* comprised the principal investigator, a junior research associate employed to work full-time on the project, and a cardiologist and a chest physician. The role of the project team was to undertake the day-to-day running of the project; this involved the identification, synthesis and interpretation of relevant evidence, the convening and running of the guideline development groups, and the production of the resulting guidelines.

The *project management group* was composed of guideline methodologists and a health informaticist; their role was to provide technical advice on a formal or informal basis throughout the project. The two *guideline development groups* were set up to undertake the task of producing the guidelines' recommendations in the light of the evidence (or its absence).

The guideline development group

Group roles and membership

The composition of a guideline development group can be considered in two ways; by the disciplines or backgrounds of the group members who would be stakeholders in the processes covered by the guideline; and by the roles required within the group. Identifying stakeholders involves identifying all the groups whose activities would be covered by the guideline or who have other legitimate reasons for having an input into the process. This is important to ensure adequate discussion of the evidence (or its absence) when developing the recommendations in the guideline.[14,15] Given that both guidelines were for use in primary care, the stakeholders involved (and their eventual numbers in each group) were as shown in Box 3.1.

From a theoretical basis we identified the roles required within the guideline development groups as those of: group member; group leader; specialist resource; technical support; and administrative support. All recruited individuals needed to have two specific characteristics: interest in the project and a positive attitude towards guidelines.

Group members were invited as individuals working in their field. Their role was to develop recommendations for practice in the light of the evidence or, if there was none, in its absence. They were not, however, expected to represent the whole range of views held within their profession.

Group leader The role of the group leader was both to ensure that the

---

Box 3.1: Guideline group members (and the eventual numbers of each)

- general practitioners (5)
- practice nurses (2 asthma, 1 angina)
- representatives of patients (1)
- secondary care physicians (1)
- public health physicians (1)
- health economist (1)
- specialist resource (1)
- small group leader (1)
- guideline methodologist (1)

---

group functioned effectively (the group process) and that it achieved its aims (the group task).[16,17] Because of the complexity of the task and the anticipated size of the group, this role was divided. A health services researcher experienced in guideline development pursued the group task for both guidelines. The other group leader supervised the group process. Group process was led by two general practitioners, external to the project team, who had considerable small group leadership experience, thus fulfilling the role of a group process leader 'whose disinterested position is unquestioned by any of the concerned parties but whose expertise in co-ordinating groups of health professionals is accepted by all'.[18]

Specialist resource   The role of specialist resource was to work with the project team to develop the literature review, perform the qualitative synthesis of the literature and to facilitate discussion of the evidence within the group meetings. These roles were fulfilled by the cardiologist and chest physician from the project team.

Technical and administrative support   Technical support was required to perform the systematic review, work with the specialist resources on its synthesis and present this to the group in a form that allowed them to make recommendations. Support was also needed to arrange external review of the draft guideline, collate reviewers' comments, feed these back to the panel, and produce the final draft of the guideline. Administrative support was required for such tasks as preparing papers for meetings, taking notes and arranging venues. Both technical and administrative roles were fulfilled by the project team.

Recruitment

Specialist resource and group leaders The specialist resources were both consultants in regional teaching hospitals. The group leaders were both experienced general practitioners (GPs) and course organisers on the local general practice vocational training scheme.

Group members were identified in a number of ways. The GPs and consultants were identified through personal knowledge or contacts of the project team. Efforts were made to enrol members from outside the North of England, although this was only successfully achieved with the asthma group to which we recruited a primary care asthma specialist who had previously been a member of a national consensus asthma guideline development panel.

It was relatively easy to identify and recruit GPs and other group members, with the exception of practice nurses and patients. Whilst there were, in a number of localities, practice nurse groups and local patient groups such as cardiac support groups, there was no regional forum for either of these groups. The practice nurses were eventually identified through personal contacts, and the patients through a community health council and a local patient support group.

As meetings were held on a weekday afternoon, group members had to have available time to commit to the work. To help overcome the difficulty of taking time out of daily work, group members were offered reimbursement of any expenditure incurred in attending the meetings, such as travel expenses and GP locum costs.

The scope of the guidelines

An important decision for the project team, subsequently endorsed by the guideline development groups, was to define the scope of the guidelines. Hadorn and Baker[1] suggest that, as cost and time are important factors in deciding a guideline's scope, there is a trade-off between depth and breadth. The narrower the scope of a guideline the more deeply a group can delve into a given area, but this is at the cost of breadth, which may leave important questions unanswered. For example, the angina group discussed whether they should restrict themselves to stable angina or include unstable angina and acute myocardial infarction, and also whether they should consider the literature on risk factor management. Whilst they acknowledged it was important to consider the management of hypertension, hypercholester-olaemia and obesity, it was explicitly agreed that systematic reviews of these areas were beyond the scope of the group; they also chose to restrict themselves to stable angina.

The identification and synthesis of evidence

Evidence review

The optimal method of evidence identification and synthesis is by systematic review.[6,15] Systematic reviews are an efficient scientific technique to identify and summarise evidence on the effectiveness of interventions that allow the generalisability and consistency of research findings to be assessed and data inconsistencies to be explored.[19] They achieve this by applying scientific principles to reduce random and systematic errors through: explicit search strategies to identify studies; explicit inclusion criteria for selecting studies for review; explicit quality assessment criteria; and rigorous methods of data abstraction and synthesis. Systematic reviews also allow the evidence in different areas of a guideline to be graded on the basis of the research design used and its susceptibility to bias.

The identification and synthesis of the literature was undertaken by the project team. Initial criteria for papers that were to be considered in the review process were that:

- they had to be published in peer-reviewed journals

- they should ideally provide evidence of effectiveness (from evalua-tions conducted under circumstances typical of routine practice), but failing this we would accept evidence of efficacy (from evaluations conducted under highly controlled circumstances not typical of routine practice)

- measures of outcome should ideally be patient-based but where these were absent intermediate, usually physiological, measures would be used

- if primary cost effectiveness studies were identified then they would be used

- studies using experimental and quasi-experimental designs (rando-mised controlled trials and both prospective and retrospective non-randomised controlled studies) would be preferred.

The search strategy A summary of the search strategies is shown in Box 3.2. While this was a pragmatic strategy influenced by the volume of papers and the time and resources available,[1] it was also felt that any new evidence that had emerged but not yet influenced practice was most likely to have been published during the previous ten years.

Box 3.2: Search strategy

- MEDLINE: 1985–94

- studies of human adults; written in English

- MeSH heading and free text searches

- search terms: meta-analysis, randomised controlled trial, reviews, cohort studies, case control studies. For asthma, we also sought the terms: asthma, peak expiratory flow rate, lung diseases obstructive, forced expiratory volume, paroxysmal dyspnoea; for stable angina the terms: coronary disease, angina pectoris

- Additional specific MEDLINE searches: decision making, theophylline, terbutaline, antihistamine, isosorbide, myocardial infarction plus secondary prevention, buccal

- BIDS electronic database, search terms: 'asthma + management', 'angina + management'.

In addition, references were identified from two other sources. First, if there was no recent evidence in a clinically important area the specialist resource was asked to identify, from his or her personal knowledge, key articles published before 1985. Second, the reference lists of non-systematic reviews were checked for relevant articles of any publication date. We did not attempt to access the grey literature, nor did we identify letters in response to original articles.

Initial sifting The identified papers were first sifted on the basis of title only by the principal investigator, a medically qualified health services researcher; they were then sifted on the basis of title and abstract by the specialist resource. Both were working to agreed criteria of clinical relevance, as the initial sift was on title alone. If there was any doubt about an article's relevance it was retained for fuller assessment.

Methodological assessment The collected papers were then assessed against a set of methodological criteria, a number of which were pass/fail.[11,12] The number of papers remaining after the various stages of the sifting process are shown in Table 3.1.

Table 3.1: Number of papers remaining after the various stages of the sifting process

Stage in the sifting process	Angina	Asthma
All references	38 675	27 401
Restricted to English language, human studies and adult subjects only	24 194	18 189
Restricted by study type	9165	4936
Sift on title alone	1810	1034
Sifted on abstract and title	699	513
Methodological screening	286	150

Clinical synthesis Papers that passed the methodological sift were then read and summarised by the specialist resource; a number of discrete areas were synthesised by other group members who were invited to take on the task. They were supported in this by members of the project team. The reviewer, with members of the project team, drew up summary evidence statements linked to the papers. The evidence was graded according to the study design using a grading system adapted from the Canadian Task Force classification[20] (*see* Table 3.2).

Table 3.2: Category of evidence

Category of evidence	Criteria
I	Well-designed randomised controlled trials, meta-analyses, or systematic reviews
II	Well-designed non-randomised prospective or retrospective controlled studies
III	Uncontrolled studies or consensus

The evidence was synthesised using qualitative methods. Quantitative (meta-analysis) techniques were not used as we were dealing with other types of studies in addition to randomised controlled trials.

The method of guideline construction

The group meetings

The groups chose to conduct their work over nine half-day meetings. The first half of the first meeting was devoted solely to introductions and discussion of the task. This latter topic recurred on a number of occasions, most frequently in the early meetings though aspects of the definition of the group task occurred all the way through. Having agreed the task the groups were presented with evidence from which they were to make recommendations. At the early meetings the groups discussed the papers and their interpretation which gave them a clear idea of the review process. As the reviewing process developed they were presented with draft recommendations linked to statements of the evidence and to blocks of summarised papers. The recommendations and the statements were then discussed and suggested changes were edited into the developing guideline by the project team between meetings. In both groups the decision-making process was informal consensus; no formal strategies were used.

Deriving recommendations

Recommendations were graded A to C as shown in Table 3.3. Both groups distinguished between the category of evidence and the strength of the associated recommendation. It was possible to have methodologically sound (category I) evidence about an area of practice that was clinically irrelevant or had such a small effect that it was of

Table 3.3: Strength of recommendation

Strength of recommendation	Criteria
A	Directly based on category I evidence
B	Directly based on category II evidence
	or extrapolated recommendation from category I evidence
C	Directly based on category III evidence
	or extrapolated recommendation from category I or II evidence

little clinical significance and would therefore attract a lower strength of recommendation. More commonly, a statement of evidence would only cover one part of an area in which a recommendation had to be made or would cover it in a way that was conflicting. Therefore, to produce a comprehensive recommendation the group had to extrapolate from the available evidence. This may lead to a strength C recommendation based upon an evidence category I statement. For example, the strength C recommendation 'short-acting beta$_2$ agonists should be used on an 'as required' basis to relieve symptoms' is supported by the evidence category I statement 'there is conflicting evidence on the issue of *prn* versus regular dosage (of short-acting beta$_2$ agonists)'. The two methodologically acceptable studies supporting the statement produced contradictory findings due to a combination of differences in patient selection, drug selection and study design (a further example of this form of grading recommendations is discussed in Chapter 7).

Areas without evidence

Both groups had to decide what to do in areas where recommendations had to be made but evidence was lacking. Limiting recommendations to areas where evidence existed would reduce the scope of the guidelines and limit their value to clinicians and policy makers who need to make decisions in the presence of imperfect knowledge.[21] The solution was to produce guidelines that contain a mixture of evidence-linked and consensus-based recommendations (RCGP, 1995).[7] The explicit grading of evidence and recommendations meant that 'areas of clinical uncertainty are demarcated . . . and a distinction made between evidence of ineffectiveness . . . and the absence of evidence for effectiveness'.[7]

The two groups chose different strategies to achieve this. The asthma group decided that in the absence of evidence their first recourse would be to a current national consensus guideline.[22] If these recommendations were appropriate they would be used. If they had been superseded, or did not provide a relevant recommendation, then the group would reach its own consensus view. In the absence of a widely recognised national guideline the angina group decided that they would make recommendations based on their experience and reach a consensus view on what the recommendation should say. Both groups agreed that if it was not possible to reach a consensus then the relevant area would be explicitly identified as one where the group could not agree. The areas without evidence generated more discussion and disagreement within the group than any of the areas in which there was evidence.

Patient involvement in guideline development

Although we invited two patients to be group members and they attended meetings regularly, they were often non-participating observers of technical discussion to which they could offer no input. While the input of patients into the process of guideline development is important, this may be better gathered outside the guideline development group, using techniques such as focus groups, rather than having a single patient as a frequently non-participating group member.

External review of the guideline

We identified the need for three groups of reviewers: guideline experts to review the methods; content area experts to review the interpretation, logic and clarity; and potential users to appraise the clinical applicability and utility of the guidelines. The purpose of the review was to identify errors in the areas that the reviewers were asked to cover; it was not to undertake a further round of consensus interpretation of the contents of the guideline. In choosing the number of reviewers there was a trade-off between the breadth of review sought and the subsequent task of dealing with detailed comments; we used up to nine reviewers on each guideline.

Reviewers' comments were amalgamated and then ordered by page of the guidelines so that they could be easily addressed by the project team and the guideline development groups to whom they were sent for written responses. All comments and responses were considered and identified errors were amended in the final draft.

Timetabling

In the original proposal to the funding body the development of the guidelines was scheduled to take 12 months; in retrospect this was not long enough. The first three months were taken up with the initial organisation of the systematic review, the identification of potential group members, and the lead time necessary before the first meetings. By the end of 12 months the nine monthly meetings of each group were complete and the draft versions of the guidelines were ready to go out to reviewers. Although reviewers were identified in advance the review process and the subsequent editing and production of the guidelines took a further six months.

There are certain fixed time periods in the process that could not be shortened. For example, once the decision had been taken to develop the guidelines over nine half-day meetings, the process inevitably took nine months because clinicians found it impossible to meet any more frequently. In addition, it would have been difficult to run the evidence review process to service a more frequent meeting schedule.

The phase that was not accurately predicted was that of external review and of the subsequent guideline production. Given the other pressures on the reviewers that we used, we were very fortunate that they felt able to offer comments within a four-week period. The collation of their comments and the responses to them required a further four weeks and these then had to be sent out to the groups for their responses with a further four-week turnaround. After further collation over the subsequent two weeks the guidelines were only then ready for the final proof-reading and production phase.

Process issues for the guideline development groups

Within the methodological process of the guideline development process there were a number of issues that affected both groups (*see* Box 3.3).

Box 3.3: What were the issues raised?

- summarising the evidence
- limitations of 'the evidence'
  - the way it is presented
  - study design
  - study end points
- making decisions
- wording recommendations

Summarising the evidence

There was clearly a large volume of evidence that had to be summarised. The groups considered the option of all group members reading all the papers but this was rejected on the grounds of the sheer volume and the group members perceived lack of both methodological and clinical expertise. However, some group members did review discrete areas supported by the project team. For most of the guideline, the groups chose the option of having the papers methodologically assessed by the project team and read for the group by the expert resource. At the first meeting of each group the expert resource was given a brief to present the evidence at each meeting as written provisional conclusions backed up with references and a summary.

Limitations of the evidence

The way evidence is presented

The problem of extracting evidence from the literature was illustrated by a quote from the consultant cardiologist when summarising papers describing randomised controlled trials of nitrate therapy:

They're badly written, badly set out . . . using 24 different exercise tests on different (drug) dosages at different times of the day.

This illustrates the technical problems of summarising evidence. We were dealing with varyingly heterogeneous studies; in the absence of being able to quantitatively combine studies this remains a fact of life for guideline developers.

Study populations

There were several problems related to the extent to which it was possible to extrapolate from the populations in studies to those that would be the subjects of guideline recommendations. For example, was it necessary to confine evidence to the disease under study: as we were developing an angina guideline could we only use drug trials in patients with angina, or could we also use evidence from studies of the same drugs in patients with hypertension? This issue also affected the groups when they were confronted with randomised controlled trials incorporating highly selective inclusion and exclusion criteria. This resulted in a trial population which was only a small subsection of the population that might come into a GP's surgery. Another example of this would be having to make recommendations for female patients when many cardiovascular studies exclude women as subjects. In the face of such restricted study populations the groups used strategies such as lowering the strength of recommendation attached to such evidence.

Two other methodological problems arose frequently. Most trials used the rate of occurrence of a defined outcome and based their power calculations on this. The guideline groups then found it difficult to interpret the data such studies presented on other, less frequent, end points, particularly if they were claiming to show no difference. This was linked to the problem of studies that failed to show a positive result yet did not have a prior power calculation; they were therefore potentially at risk, by being too small and failing to detect an effect that was actually present.

The final example of methodological problems that limited the usefulness of evidence was that of trials apparently comparing two drugs. Some studies merely simultaneously compared two preparations each against placebo and then drew conclusions about their relative effectiveness, usually claiming they were as good as each other, without ever having directly compared them. In addition, patients were maintained on background therapy that was often poorly described.

Study end points

There was a mismatch between the factors on which group members wanted to make decisions and those that were available. A GP said:

many of the drug trials don't actually measure the sort of end points that you might actually want to know about.

They wanted to make recommendations based on information about quality of life or increased life expectancy; studies usually used intermediate end points such as increased exercise time on a treadmill; or an increased peak flow. In the absence of a known direct link between such intermediate measures and those on which the group wanted information such evidence was felt to be of limited value.

Making decisions

The process of decision making was explored in an exercise by one of the groups (see Box 3.4). The purpose of the exercise was to illustrate that such decision making was usually implicit and was influenced by assumptions, beliefs and values with little in the way of evidence involved in the process.

Box 3.4: Decision-making exercise

- You have won both the holiday and the car of your dreams.
- However, you have to leave on the holiday in three hours' time and the car has to be bought before you return.
- You have to tell somebody how to buy the car that you want.

Within the guideline development process decisions were, not surprisingly, more difficult when assumptions, beliefs or values were challenged, either by the evidence or in its absence. Group members seemed happier to have their beliefs challenged by evidence on the basis that this was something they could now accept that they had not previously known. However, the absence of evidence prompted much debate. In the asthma group, one group member quite firmly stated that all patients presenting to GPs with a possible diagnosis of asthma should have a chest X-ray; there was no evidence around this and no one else in the group agreed. The group dealt with this by identifying it as a potential issue for future research; they did not recommend routine chest X-ray in the investigation of newly presenting wheezing patients.

Wording recommendations

Both groups dealt at some length with the issue of wording of recommendations; the issue became to what extent recommendations should be seen as potentially flexible or rigid and this was reflected in the use of terms such as 'must do' as opposed to 'should' or 'could do'. To deal with this a 'qualifying paragraph' was included within the introduction of the guidelines (*see* Box 3.5).

Box 3.5: 'Qualifying paragraph' from the guidelines

The development group assumes that healthcare professionals will use general medical knowledge and clinical judgement in applying the general principles and specific recommendations of this document to the management of individual patients. Recommendations may not be appropriate for use in all circumstances. Decisions to adopt any particular recommendation must be made by the practitioner in the light of available resources and circumstances presented by individual patients.

Where the evidence was strong, firmer recommendations were drawn and more compelling terms were used, such as 'should'. This was done in the belief that this reflected the development groups' views yet allowed a practitioner to interpret it in the light of the 'qualifying paragraph'. Where evidence was weak or absent, recommendations were worded in a more permissive style using words such as 'could' or 'might'.

Conclusion

Guideline development requires a range of skills. Identifying and assimilating the evidence required the skills of systematic reviewing to identify relevant papers and then the skills of an experienced and critical clinician to summarise their clinical relevance. The evidence was fed into large multidisciplinary groups that needed skilled leadership to ensure the groups both worked effectively and achieved their tasks. The product of the groups' deliberations had to be turned into an evidence-based guideline. This range of skills is central to the successful development of any guideline that requires *de novo* evidence review.

The issues that we have presented are central to the development of valid guidelines but practical experience of dealing with these issues is very limited in the UK and we present our experiences as a first step in understanding how these issues affect evidence-based guideline development within the NHS. Methodological expertise needs to be developed at both national and local levels and resources need to be committed to the process. It is only by investing in such processes that the validity of the guideline can be optimised.[5]

References

1 Hadorn DC and Baker D (1994) Development of the AHCPR-sponsored heart failure guideline: methodologic and procedural issues. *Journal on Quality Improvement*, **20**: 539–47.

2 Woolf SH (1992) Practice guidelines – a new reality in medicine: II. Methods of developing guidelines. *Archives of Internal Medicine*, **152**: 946–52.

3 Agency for Health Care Policy and Research (1992). *Acute Pain Management: Operative or Medical Procedures and Trauma*. AHCPR/ US Department of Health and Human Services, Rockville, MD.

4 Agency for Health Care Policy and Research (1994) *Heart Failure: Management of Patients with Left Ventricular Systolic Dysfunction*.

AHCPR/US Department of Health and Human Services, Rockville, MD.

5   Field MJ and Lohr KN (eds) (1992) *Guidelines for Clinical Practice: From Development To Use.* Institute of Medicine/National Academy Press, Washington DC.

6   Grimshaw JM, Eccles MP and Russell IT (1995) Developing clinically valid practice guidelines. *Journal of Evaluation in Clinical Practice*, **1**: 37–48.

7   Royal College of General Practitioners (1995) *The Development and Implementation of Clinical Guidelines: Report of the Clinical Guidelines Working Group.* Report from Practice 26. RCGP, Exeter.

8   Eccles MP, Clapp Z, Grimshaw JM, Adams PC, Higgins B, Purves I and Russell IT (1996) *North of England Evidence Based Guideline Development Project: Methods of Guideline Development. BMJ*, **312**: 760–1.

9   North of England Asthma Guideline Development Project (1996) Summary version of evidence based guideline for the primary care management of asthma in adults. *BMJ*, **312**: 762–6.

10 North of England Stable Angina Guideline Development Group (1996) Summary version of evidence based guideline for the primary care management of stable angina in adults. *BMJ*, **312**: 827–32.

11 North of England Evidence Based Guideline Development Project (1996) *Evidence Based Clinical Practice Guideline: The Primary Care Management of Stable Angina.* Report No. 74. Centre for Health Services Research, Newcastle-upon-Tyne.

12 North of England Evidence Based Guideline Development Project (1996) *Evidence Based Clinical Practice Guideline: The Primary Care Management of Asthma in Adults.* Report No. 75. Centre for Health Services Research, Newcastle-upon-Tyne.

13 Secretary of State for Health (1992) *The Health of the Nation: A Strategy for Health in England.* HMSO, London.

14 Russell IT, Grimshaw JM and Wilson B (1993) Scientific and methodological issues in quality assurance. In: JS Beck, IAD Bouchier and IT Russell (eds) *Quality Assurance in Medical Care.* Edinburgh: Proceedings of the Royal Society of Edinburgh, **101B**: 77–103.

15 Grimshaw JM and Russell IT (1993) Achieving health gain through clinical guidelines. I. Developing scientifically valid guidelines. *Quality in Health Care*, **2**: 243–8.

16 Scott M and Marinker ML (1990) Small group work. In ML Marinker (ed) *Medicine Audit and General Practice.* London, British Medical Journal Publications.

17 Newton JC, Hutchinson A, Steen IN, Russell IT and Haines EV (1992) Educational potential of medical audit: observations from a study of small groups setting standards. *Quality in Health Care*, **1**: 256–9.

18 Park RE, Fink A, Brook RH, Chassin MR, Kahn KL, Merrick NJ *et al.* (1986) Physician ratings of appropriate indications for six medical and surgical procedures. *American Journal Public Health*, **76**: 766–72.

19 Mulrow CD (1994) Systematic review: rationale for systematic reviews. *BMJ*, **309**: 597–9.

20 Canadian Task Force (1979) Task Force classification of study designs. *Canadian Medical Association Journal*, **121**: 1193–254

21 Lomas J (1993) Making clinical policy explicit: legislative policy making and lessons for developing practice guidelines. *International Journal for Technological Assessment in Health Care*, **9**: 11–25.

22 British Thoracic Society, British Paediatric Association, Royal College of Physicians, King's Fund Centre, National Asthma Campaign, Royal College of General Practitioners, General Practitioners in Asthma Group, British Association of Accident and Emergency Medicine, and British Paediatric Respiratory Group (1993) Guidelines on the management of asthma. *Thorax*, **48**: 1–24.

Acknowledgement

This chapter is based on an article originally published in *Quality in Health Care* (1996), **5**: 44–50, and has been published with the permission of the authors and British Medical Journal Publishing Group.

4
Development of multiprofessional guidelines for cardiac rehabilitation: a survey-based approach

David Thompson and Alison Kitson

Although there is a growing consensus on the methods of developing evidence-based guidelines, the approaches for including empirical data on current practice are less clear-cut. Multidisciplinary workshops have often been used to achieve a measure of agreement among multiprofessional groups, usually supported by evidence from published literature. In the case of the national cardiac rehabilitation guidelines, a survey of current practice was used as an additional means of identifying the important clinical areas to be addressed by the guideline. Here, the authors describe some of the strengths and weaknesses of this triangulated approach. By combining four methods: evidence reviewing, consensus development, surveying the organisation of cardiac rehabilitation care nationally, and developing clinical audit tools, they seek to bridge the gap between guideline development and implementation of recommendations.

Introduction

Clinical guidelines are aids to, not substitutes for, clinical judgement[1] and are powerful tools for helping to get research evidence into practice and as such are an important part of any clinical effectiveness initiative.[2,3]

The recent document *A First Class Service: Quality in the New NHS*[4] sets out the government's aim to place quality at the heart of healthcare. National standards will be set through National Service Frameworks and through the National Institute for Clinical Excellence (NICE). NICE will produce clear guidance for clinicians about which treatments work for which patients, including among other things, clinical guidelines.

Cardiac rehabilitation is a field in which a number of complex interventions, delivered by a range of healthcare professionals, may take place, some of which are supported by robust evidence, some by expert opinion and others of which are even more questionable. The challenge is to develop a system to pull this information together. This chapter, therefore, describes the construction of a national guideline for cardiac rehabilitation, and outlines choices clinicians have to make about how they agree best practice in the absence of evidence.

Cardiac rehabilitation services are much more developed and more widely offered in the US than in the UK. A major aim of the UK cardiac rehabilitation guideline was to encourage a standard of service across the country that would offer access to all patients who are likely to benefit. This national guideline would serve as a basis for locally developed guidelines and further research.

What is 'cardiac rehabilitation?

Box 4.1: The World Health Organisation definition of cardiac rehabilitation[5]

. . . the sum of activities required to influence favourably the underlying cause of the disease, as well as to ensure the patients the best possible physical, mental and social conditions so that they may, by their own efforts, preserve, or resume when lost, as normal a place as possible in the life of the community. Rehabilitation cannot be regarded as an isolated form of therapy, but must be integrated with the whole treatment, of which it forms only one facet. (p 5)

The World Health Organisation definition of cardiac rehabilitation is shown in Box 4.1. It is, of course, all-embracing but is still endorsed by countries in Europe and beyond. In essence, cardiac rehabilitation services are comprehensive programmes involving education, exercise, risk factor modification and counselling, designed to limit the physiological and psychological effects of heart disease, reduce the risk of death or recurrence of the cardiac event and enhance the psychosocial and vocational state of patients.

A British Cardiac Society working party report[6] recommended that every district hospital which treats patients with heart disease should provide a cardiac rehabilitation service, and that individual programmes should evaluate their outcome, and a standard format of audit could be agreed nationally to allow comparison. However, the Audit Commission[7] pointed out that the provision of cardiac rehabilitation is still a neglected topic in some districts and hospitals.

Guidelines for cardiac rehabilitation

Although there is some scepticism, particularly among cardiologists, regarding the effectiveness of cardiac rehabilitation, there is strong evidence attesting to its benefit.[8] Authoritative bodies, such as the Agency for Health Care Policy and Research (AHCPR),[9] which published an evidence-based guideline on the same topic in 1995, have concluded that there is sufficient evidence available to demonstrate substantial benefits (*see* Box 4.2).

Box 4.2: Benefits of cardiac rehabilitation[9] (with strength of evidence A to D)	
• improvement in exercise tolerance	A
• improvement in symptoms	B
• improvement in blood lipid levels	B
• reduction in cigarette smoking	B
• improvement in psychosocial well-being and reduction of stress	A

The AHCPR guidelines, developed simultaneously with the UK guidelines, adopted a more systematic and rigorous approach, supported as they were by greater funding and resources. However, in essence, the final recommendations were very similar.

Cardiac rehabilitation guidelines have been available in the US for some years and are regularly updated. For example, in 1991, the American Association of Cardiovascular and Pulmonary Rehabilitation (AACPR) produced the first set of guidelines for practising cardiac rehabilitation.[10] The second edition, published in 1995, substantially updated and expanded upon the first edition.[11]

The AACPR clinical guideline, based on a critical review of 400 scientific papers, highlights the major effects (see above) of multifactorial cardiac rehabilitation services on physical and psychosocial recovery of patients with coronary heart disease (CHD) and following cardiac surgery. The guideline informs clinicians about what outcomes may be achieved through specific interventions and notes limitations in the available evidence. However, the guideline was not published until late 1995, and therefore was not available at the time of the development of the UK guidelines.

Constructing a guideline for cardiac rehabilitation

The work described is based on the experience of the authors who, representing the Royal College of Nursing and collaborating with colleagues from the Royal College of Physicians and the British Cardiac Society, were asked by the Department of Health in England to construct a guideline for cardiac rehabilitation in 1994. The study comprised four phases, which attempted to triangulate evidence from the literature, current practice and professional opinion as unstructured consensus (see Box 4.3).

Box 4.3: Phases of the guideline development

1 Literature review of the evidence for cardiac rehabilitation.
2 Postal survey of centres in England and Wales offering cardiac rehabilitation.
3 In-depth study of current practice in a random sample of centres.
4 Workshop on the preparation of guidelines and audit standards.

Literature review

The strategy for searching the literature for the review was based on the standard practice, although necessarily limited to only three main library databases because of limited resources (*see* Box 4.4).

Box 4.4: The literature search

- MEDLINE and CINAHL searches were accessed via CD-ROM and a free-text search using Thesaurus was undertaken
- BIDS search was also undertaken
- MeSH terms were used and the search strategy was commenced from 1983 to identify literature over the previous ten years
- the research strategy was augmented through secondary searches of references that were provided by the articles thus identified, as well as those culled from review articles
- recognised national and international experts in cardiac rehabilitation were solicited for appropriate literature citations.

Cardiac rehabilitation services tend to draw on a broad spectrum of techniques and professionals, have an equally broad conceptual base and depend crucially on the input of patients. In order to determine the research base pertaining to cardiac rehabilitation, it was therefore essential to undertake an extensive review of the relevant published literature relating to nine areas of clinical importance:

1 exercise training

2 education

3 counselling

4 behavioural interventions

5 risk assessment and stratification

6 adherence (compliance)

7 cost and cost-effectiveness

8 secondary prevention

9 quality of life.

The search strategy yielded around 800 articles, of which less than one-third could be considered to be relevant in that they addressed elements of cardiac rehabilitation. Preference was given to research reports using a randomised controlled study design, although it was acknowledged that a poorly designed and executed trial may be less reliable than other types of study. Four meta-analyses of the effectiveness of cardiac rehabilitation interventions were also identified. Thus the literature review reaffirmed one of the difficulties for guideline developers. If randomised controlled trials are seen as the 'gold standard' for evidence, then less weight is inevitably placed by evidence grading systems on cohort studies, large audit projects and well-designed qualitative studies. Yet, in some circumstances these may be the most valuable means of answering important questions. Further development on evidence grading for guidelines remains a priority. Studies reporting findings in the psychological, educational and social literature were often of a qualitative nature, whereas those related to exercise were more often of a quantitative nature. Nevertheless, interpretation of benefit in studies is complicated by the variety of outcome measures used and the time that they are obtained despite what appears to be an extensive literature.

Because cardiac rehabilitation is often a multifaceted intervention, it can be difficult to ascertain whether benefits, if they accrue, are due to a single component or a combination of components. It may be that some interaction of factors is responsible, in other words, the whole of the intervention is more than the sum of the parts. In addition, although cardiac rehabilitation often begins around six weeks after the cardiac event and usually continues for at least two months, the lifestyle changes recommended to many patients will not have a significant impact on their health state for many months or even years. Adherence to treatment regimes is therefore a problem, causing 'drop-out' from trials and studies with consequent loss of power.

Review of current practice

In parallel with the literature review the project set out to identify the extent and variation in current cardiac rehabilitation practice, with two purposes. First, to assist in refining the clinical problems the guidelines should address. Secondly, to ensure the guideline focused on issues where clinical variation was apparent. Context of the health service – who was doing what and where – was seen as important information by which to shape the guideline.

A preliminary postal survey conducted in 1994 identified 199 centres in England and Wales which offered cardiac rehabilitation services. Twenty-five of these centres were subsequently chosen at random for a site visit by a member of the research team in order to determine the nature and extent of cardiac rehabilitation service provision.[12] The survey found wide variation in resources available for the rehabilitation of CHD patients. Three-quarters of the centres had commenced their programmes within the previous five years, usually at the instigation of interested staff. There were often restrictions on entry; elderly people were excluded in ten centres, women only represented 15% of attendees, and patients with more complex cardiac problems, such as angina and heart failure, were under-represented.

The central components of all programmes were education and exercise training but there was a wide range in the quantity and quality of service provision. Little was available in the way of choice; most programmes were hospital out-patient based, staffing varied and nearly one-third had no identifiable funding.[13] From this survey it was clear that guidelines were needed to offer a framework for this service that had rapidly expanded in recent years.

Developing the guideline

Following the convention for guideline development at that time,[14] a workshop was convened under the auspices of the Royal College of Nursing, Royal College of Physicians, and the British Cardiac Society in order to construct a national guideline and audit standards for cardiac rehabilitation which would be made available to commissioners and providers (and to general practitioners who are taking an increasing role in commissioning healthcare). The aim of the consensus workshop was to present the evidence available, derived from the literature review and the survey of current practice, and to gain agreement on recommendations distilled from these two sources of information.

This process was undertaken by identifying key clinicians and researchers in the field of cardiac rehabilitation who were invited to prepare and present background papers at the workshop. The object was to review the literature in relation to a specific aspect of cardiac rehabilitation and prepare a concise but informative report summarising the research evidence available and making a number of key recommendations. Eight aspects were identified (see Box 4.5). The eight background papers were circulated to each participant one month before

---

Box 4.5: Cardiac rehabilitation: the key recommendations

1 *Needs and action priorities*	e.g. people with heart failure should be included since they have a high chance of health benefit
2 *Medical component*	e.g. risk–benefit important in defining high risk subgroups
3 *Psychological component*	e.g. use a simple formal assessment for anxiety/depression pre-discharge
4 *Social component*	e.g. strong partner support possibly strongest factor in buffering disruption of relationships at home/work/social groups
5 *Exercise component*	e.g. patients with myocardial infarction (MI), unstable angina or heart failure should have a recorded assessment of exercise capacity before hospital discharge
6 *Vocational component*	e.g. between 62 and 92% of patients who were working before MI will return to work after rehabilitation
7 *Economic component*	e.g. medical costs are marginally lower and patient income greater in patients who participate in rehabilitation programmes
8 *Patients' experiences*[15]	e.g. patients report cardiac rehabilitation to be helpful

---

the workshop. The composition of the workshop was judged to be an important consideration and 19 people took part representing consumers and health and social care professions, including:

- cardiology
- exercise physiology
- general medicine
- general practice
- health economics

- health psychology
- medical sociology
- nursing
- occupational therapy
- physiotherapy
- psychiatry
- rehabilitation medicine.

The participants also represented a variety of professional Royal Colleges, allied organisations and charities. At the workshop, the main points from each of the papers were presented by the author after which an opportunity for full discussion was offered to all those present. The proceedings were audiotaped and transcribed throughout and subsequently produced as a report which was sent to each participant (*see* Box 4.6). Ultimately, agreement with no substantive changes was confirmed for the guideline and audit points, which were then published with everyone's approval.[16]

Box 4.6: Five stages of the guideline development

1 Experts identified and invited to prepare background papers
↓
2 Background papers circulated to participants
↓
3 Workshop convened
↓
4 Background papers presented and discussed
↓
5 Report of guideline confirmed

The content of the cardiac rehabilitation guideline, with examples of recommendations, is shown in Box 4.7.

Box 4.7: Content and examples of recommendations in the guideline

- *Process of care* (e.g. spanning the time course of cardiac rehabilitation are three essential elements: explanation and understanding, specific rehabilitation interventions, and re-adaptation and re-education).

- *Scope of rehabilitation entry criteria* (e.g. patients with heart failure, valvular heart disease, angina, and hypertension may have a large potential for health gain and could be helped by targeted rehabilitation programmes).

- *Components* (e.g. medical diagnosis and intervention, psycho-social care, exercise, education and vocational assessment).

- *Cost-effectiveness* (e.g. proper cost-effectiveness assessments of integrated rehabilitation programmes are urgently needed).

- *Setting* (e.g. responsibility for phase I (in hospital) rehabilitation rested with everyone who dealt with or treated cardiac patients, whether in hospital or a cardiac setting, phase II (early post-discharge) and phase III (later post-discharge) rehabilitation requires facilities that are best provided and co-ordinated at secondary level, and phase IV (long-term follow-up) rehabilitation falls largely within the primary care setting).

- *Clinical standards* (e.g. patients should routinely be assessed for risk factors as part of in-patient or out-patient management, and clear advice given on risk factor correction).

- *Contracting* (e.g. commissioner/provider agreements need to specify the scope of the agreement, such as all cardiac diagnoses or selected diagnoses, whether access will be open or limited to hospital referrals).

Development of an audit tool

The material gathered from the workshop also contributed to the development of a cardiac rehabilitation audit tool[17] (*see* Box 4.8). Information was converted into simple statements that were clear and unambiguous, would obtain useful information that was easily access-ible, and could be used by a range of health service personnel to assess the quality of their care. The main principles in constructing the tool were to: address important cardiac rehabilitation issues; design a clear

---

Box 4.8: The audit tool

- *Initiating event* (e.g. angina, MI, cardiac surgery).
- *Risk factor assessment* (e.g. do the notes contain a record of blood pressure?).
- *Exercise capacity* (e.g. do the notes contain a record of the patient having an exercise test?).
- *Personal plan* (e.g. do the notes contain a record of the patient being given a written personal rehabilitation plan?).
- *Exercise programme* (e.g. do the notes contain a record of exercise advice?).
- *Psychological state* (e.g. do the notes contain a record of a formal assessment of anxiety and depression?).
- *Education and support* (e.g. do the notes contain a record of whether the patient and partner have been offered education?).
- *Medical investigations and treatment* (e.g. do the notes contain a record of whether the patient is receiving aspirin?).

---

and concise format no longer than one page of A4; seek information that should be readily available to enable the recording of information that was likely to lead to improvements in the quality of care; and enable completion by any health professional.

After compilation, the audit proformas were reviewed by some of the workshop participants and amendments were made following their advice. This process was repeated until agreed proformas emerged and were ready for testing. The testing took place in three cardiac rehabilitation centres and following some refinement the guideline was made available by the Royal College of Physicians.

Dissemination and implementation of the guideline

Although the development of the guideline was funded by the Department of Health, dissemination and implementation were not. The risk was that poor dissemination of the guideline would be likely to lessen any impact and reduce the chances of achieving the primary aim of improving the quality of cardiac rehabilitation services. In fact, this risk has been recognised in UK national guidelines projects. For instance, in the Scottish Intercollegiate Guideline programme (SIGN), substantial resources are given to disseminating a programme of guidelines. In this case, although health service funding was not available for dissemination, as the guideline had been produced under the auspices of the Royal College of Nursing, the Royal College of Physicians and the British Cardiac Society, legitimacy was afforded to them by individuals and organisations associated with cardiac rehabilitation. Furthermore the British Heart Foundation and the British Association for Cardiac Rehabilitation endorsed the guideline and subsequently supported the publication of an edited and updated version of the background review papers presented at a workshop.[18]

Whether this endorsement will have an impact on the implementation and rate of uptake of the guideline is unknown. A pilot study concerned with the implementation of the guideline has been undertaken which compared three cardiac rehabilitation settings: those actively receiving guidelines and additional facilitation; those actively receiving guidelines; and those not actively receiving guidelines. The findings[19] showed that the guideline did not appear to have been utilised, other than having been mentioned in brief discussions. This suggests that although the guideline is endorsed by key bodies the real challenge is still implementation. Successful implementation of the guideline will include organisational and managerial aspects and systems for their audit and evaluation, and this should ideally take place alongside local quality improvement strategies.[20]

Lessons learnt

The development of clinical guidelines is a rapidly growing industry and although the approach taken by the authors in the construction of this guideline seemed appropriate at the time, it is clear, with hindsight, that it has a number of limitations and lessons to learn. The aim was to produce explicit recommendations that were both scientifically valid and helpful in clinical practice, but it was clear that there would have to be a degree of pragmatism in the assembling of information and the construction of the guideline.[21, 22] Financial and time constraints imposed by the funding agency further limited the scope of the project. More recent national guideline projects have sought funding to review systematically and weight the evidence, with consequent increases in cost. The method of construction was certainly not as sophisticated as that since adopted by others; however, there were good reasons at the time why it was not. First, cardiac rehabilitation is a rather complex and relatively under-researched intervention and there is a dearth of hard scientific evidence, particularly randomised controlled trials. So, the guidelines were constructed on the best evidence available at that time as well expert clinical judgement. When the scientific literature was incomplete or inconsistent, the guidelines reflected the professional judgement of experts. This approach may have resulted in reliance on the group's knowledge of published work and their own clinical experiences, and it is acknowledged that an incomplete literature search strategy may result in important findings being missed and a degree of selection bias. Although the guideline reflects the state of knowledge at the time of publication, given the inevitable changes in the state of scientific information and technology, periodic review, updating and revision will be necessary.

Inexperience in this form of professional collaboration placed limits on what was achievable. Cardiac rehabilitation is very much about multidisciplinary team work. To reach agreement amongst a rich variety of users and providers of cardiac rehabilitation services was never going to be an easy task and difficulties of developing multiprofessional guidelines have been addressed recently.[23] Each individual, whether representing themselves, their discipline or an organisation, would have their own different views, priorities and agendas. This was especially true among the physicians (two cardiologists, a general practitioner, a general physician and two rehabilitation physicians) who had difficulty agreeing on certain clinical cardiological issues and the interpretation or weighting that should be placed on specific pieces of research evidence. In Chapter 5, McIntosh reviews methods which might now be used to improve the value of consensus building in guideline development.

Conclusion

In the approach described in this chapter, the development of multi-professional guidelines has demonstrated some of the strengths and weaknesses of what might be called the pragmatic approach. Limitation of resources can lead to methods which are open to critisism, yet in reality produce a product which may still be useful, provided the limitations are presented explicitly. Contrasts between approaches taken in Chapters 2, 3 and 4 also demonstrate how quickly the methods on guideline development have changed, with an increasing methodological rigour being demanded sometimes when guideline projects have already agreed, fixed budgets. The lessons learnt here may prove valuable for those intending to embark on a similar excercise.

References

1   Field MJ and Lohr KN (eds) (1992) *Guidelines for Clinical Practice: From Development to Use.* Institute of Medicine/National Academy Press, Washington DC.

2   Kitson AL (1995) The multi-professional agenda and clinical effectiveness. In: MT Deighan and S Hitch (eds) *Clinical Effectiveness: From Guidelines to Cost Effective Practice.* HMSO, London.

3   National Health Service Executive (1996) *Promoting Clinical Effectiveness. A Framework for Action In and Through the NHS.* NHS Executive, Leeds.

4   Department of Health (1998) *A First Class Service: Quality in the New NHS.* HMSO, London.

5   World Health Organisation (1993) *Needs and Action Priorities in Cardiac Rehabilitation and Secondary Prevention in Patients with CHD.* WHO Regional Office for Europe, Copenhagen.

6   Horgan J, Bethell H, Carson P *et al.* (1992) Working party report on cardiac rehabilitation. *British Heart Journal,* **67**: 412–18.

7   Audit Commission (1995) *Dear to Our Hearts? Commissioning Services for the Treatment and Prevention of Coronary Heart Disease.* HMSO, London.

8   Thompson DR and Bowman GS (1997) Evidence for the effectiveness of cardiac rehabilitation. *Clinical Effectiveness in Nursing,* **1**: 64–75.

9   Wenger NK, Froelicher ES, Smith LK *et al.* (1995) *Cardiac Rehabilitation.* Clinical Practice Guideline No. 17. US Department of Health and Human Services, Public Health Service, Agency for Health Care Policy and Research and the National, Heart, Lung, and Blood Institute, Rockville, MD.

10 American Association of Cardiovascular and Pulmonary Rehabilitation (1991) *Guidelines for Cardiac Rehabilitation Programs.* Human Kinetics, Champaign, IL.

11 American Association of Cardiovascular and Pulmonary Rehabilitation (1995) *Guidelines for Cardiac Rehabilitation Programs.* Human Kinetics, Champaign, IL.

12 Thompson DR, Bowman GS, Kitson AL *et al.* (1997) Cardiac rehabilitation services in England and Wales: a national survey. *International Journal of Cardiology,* **59**: 299–304.

13 Gray AM, Bowman GS and Thompson DR (1997) The cost of cardiac rehabilitation services in England and Wales. *Journal of the Royal College of Physicians of London,* **31**: 57–61.

14 Lomas J (1993) Making clinical policy explicit. Legislative policy making and lessons for developing practice guidelines. *International Journal of Technology Assessment in Health Care*, **9**: 11–25.

15 Duff LA, Kelson M, Marriott S *et al.* (1996) Clinical guidelines: involving patients and users of services. *Journal of Clinical Effectiveness*, **1**: 104–12.

16 Thompson DR, Bowman GS, Kitson AL *et al.* (1996) Cardiac rehabilitation in the United Kingdom: guidelines and audit standards. *Heart*, **75**: 89–93.

17 Thompson DR, Bowman GS, de Bono DP *et al.* (1997) The development and testing of a cardiac rehabilitation audit tool. *Journal of the Royal College of Physicians of London*, **31**: 161–4.

18 Thompson DR, Bowman GS, de Bono DP *et al.* (eds) (1997) *Cardiac Rehabilitation: Guidelines and Audit Standards.* Royal College of Physicians, London.

19 Stokes HC, Thompson DR and Seers K (1998) The implementation of multi-professional guidelines for cardiac rehabilitation: a pilot study. *Coronary Health Care*, **2**: 60–71.

20 Duff L, Kitson AL, Seers K and Humphris D (1996) Clinical guidelines: an introduction to their development and implementation. *Journal of Advanced Nursing*, **23**: 887–95.

21 Grimshaw J and Russell I (1993) Achieving health gain through clinical guidelines: 1. Developing scientifically valid guidelines. *Quality in Health Care*, **2**: 243–8.

22 Grimshaw J and Russell I (1993) Achieving health gain through clinical guidelines: II. Ensuring guidelines change medical practice. *Quality in Health Care*, **3**: 45–52.

23 Wray J and Maresh M (1997) Multi-professional guidelines: can we move beyond tribal boundaries? *Quality in Health Care*, **6**: 57–8.

5
Guidance: what role should consensus play in guideline development?

Aileen McIntosh

Developing guidelines is not a purely objective process; there is still a great deal of subjectivity involved at different stages of the development process. This subjectivity arises because of the inadequacy of evidence to address many clinical questions that practitioners want answered and that guidelines try to address. It also is sometimes introduced by the political nature of much guideline development. This chapter looks at the use of consensus in guideline development, particularly in the process of moving from evidence statements to the derivation of recommendations. Using experience from North America and from the recent development of national clinical guidelines in the UK, the author examines the relationship between subjectivity, consensus development and the pressure to produce evidence-based guidelines. The role of subjectivity in guideline development is discussed, as is the relationship between subjectivity and the consequent need for consensus building.

Introduction: the dilemma of relying only on scientific evidence

There is growing acceptance that clinical practice should accord with principles derived from rigorous studies of effectiveness. At the same time there is also recognition, and a degree of acceptance, that this evidence-based approach cannot adequately deal with all aspects of clinical practice. As Woolf and colleagues[1] have argued:

There are important limitations to the evidence-based approach, however, beginning with the shortage of good data. Proof of effectiveness is lacking for most of what is done in medicine . . .

. . . clinical practice would come to a halt if practitioners could only perform tests and treatments that had been proven effective in clinical trials. (p 514)

Thus, clinical practice goes on using evidence as a basis when it is available and tradition, opinion and perceptions of what constitutes current good practice when it is not.

Even in areas where evidence is available and substantial, it is not always the case that it is in agreement and unidirectional. Not uncommonly, this may mean that practice based on evidence is not clearly defined, with the result that disagreement and divergence about what practice should be followed continues to exist. Thus, in both areas where evidence is and is not available it is often the case, as Skrabanek[2] observed, that:

the very need for consensus stems from a lack of consensus. (p 1446)

Yet, summaries of evidence are considered useful, indeed increasingly necessary, to help practitioners manage, and understand, the ever burgeoning research evidence base. They can help practitioners locate relevant evidence, and evidence-linked guidelines are a further example of tools that can help practitioners navigate their way through the maze of research information.

Subjectivity in guideline development

The opportunities for subjectivity to intrude into a seemingly objective guideline development process are myriad, occurring at all stages in development, from topic selection, development and framing of questions to be addressed, evidence reviewing through to the drafting of final recommendations. Topic selection for guideline development is unlikely to be purely objective since personal and organisational agendas intrude. Nor is the decision process that determines the scope of the guideline wholly objective for very similar reasons.

As Eccles and colleagues demonstrate in Chapter 3, the processes of identifying, selecting and sifting evidence are based on a series of decisions – all of which provide the opportunity to involve subjectivity. The process is designed to be as objective as possible. But if it were always so then there would always be perfect inter-rater reliability between reviewers in choice of study for inclusion in evidence reviews – and this is not the case. The process of turning evidence statements into recommendations is the main area of concern in this discussion, as this is at the heart of the process of producing clinical guidelines and is what makes guidelines essentially different from systematic reviews and other types of evidence summaries.

It is almost inconceivable that subjectivity will not enter into the process of turning evidence statements into recommendations. Evidence statements are reports of what the scientific evidence states in particular areas; they are not usually statements of action. Rather, they are in essence passive reports of scientific findings. Hence, a series of evidence statements does not equate to a set of recommendations and guidelines.

Clinical guideline recommendations, on the other hand, *are* statements suggesting particular actions. Therefore, to turn (passive) evidence statements into (active) recommendations, further stages of a development and interpretative process need to be undergone. Without this process, the collection of evidence statements remains a summary of evidence, and not a guideline. Therefore, a key requirement in the guideline is clarity so that users can see what is an evidence statement and what is a recommendation.

The process of incorporating evidence and opinion into guideline development is not easy, nor are the methods straightforward. As Shekelle and Shriger[3] point out:

There is little guidance on the optimum way to mix expert opinion with scientific literature. (p 1)

In many instances of guideline development, the available evidence may not help to answer questions of clinical practice and in most instances this shortfall is addressed by the use of clinical opinion. Leape and colleagues[4] argue:

Because of the inevitable incompleteness of scientific data, any process to develop comprehensive guidelines for the use of procedures must combine data with opinion. (p 152)

Moreover, this synthesis of evidence and opinion is a process that has to be undertaken even in guidelines that are predominantly evidence-based. The process of taking research findings and turning them into recommendations involves mixing scientific evidence with the views of the guideline development panel. Thus the process involves a degree of subjectivity, as Fletcher and colleagues[5] point out:

Expert opinion is incorporated into all practice guidelines, and even evidence-based groups are forced to make subjective judgements about the quality of evidence or its generalizability to clinical practice. (p 2009)

Recommendations may be derived from strong or weak evidence bases. As a result, the development group might wish to assign a higher or lower recommendation grading than the weight of the evidence base might suggest. This may be the result of discussion about the clinical significance of a particular intervention or issue. For example, there may be an important element of clinical practice for which there is little or no evidence about the most effective interventions or there may be no evidence because research has not been conducted in that area, or any research conducted has been of such poor quality that it is not possible to draw any conclusions about effectiveness. Thus, the usual argument would be that the poor evidence base would mean that any recommendations offered in that area would have a low grading.

Nevertheless, the development group might want to make a strong recommendation, with a high grading, because it is such an important clinical area. If this were done then the guideline user could reasonably expect a full explanation and description of the process that underlies that decision. Thus, the decision-making process, outlining the relative role of evidence and the considerable degree of discussion and consensus that are combined to derive a recommendation, should be available for scrutiny by the guideline user.

Similarly, consideration of different types of evidence, is in itself a subjective decision process and subjectivity is increasingly evident when considering non-RCT (randomised controlled trial) evidence. Where evidence is available but contradictory, then, subjectivity potentially plays an even more significant part in recommendation derivation.

The nature of evidence for guidelines

Current methods of evidence assessment have RCTs as their starting point, and usually as their 'gold standard'. But the assessment of trial evidence is not yet perfected, and the means of appropriately assessing non-trial evidence have hardly begun to be addressed. Given that most healthcare is not about a particular pharmacological intervention, then it is likely that most healthcare issues are perhaps not most appropriately addressed by RCTs. So, guideline developers need help, as do other practitioners of evidence-based healthcare, in being able to assess, accurately and effectively, the many other forms of evidence other than RCTs. Until then subjectivity comes into many aspects of using evidence to form the basis of recommendations.

Answering questions

One of the particular issues for guideline developers in deriving evidence-based recommendations is that the evidence may not be in the same areas as the clinical questions to which practitioners need answers. The evidence base may not address the questions which clinicians have, and the evidence base may not have been constructed in a way that addresses, or can be used to address, these clinical questions. Therefore, even in areas where evidence exists, its utility for guideline developers may be limited.

Where evidence is not available, then the subjective process of arriving at any recommendation is usually based on professional opinion, experience, assumptions, beliefs and judgement, a situation faced by Thompson and Kitson in Chapter 4. Given that these recommendations are subjective, individualistic, potentially biased and more prone to interpretation and inaccuracy, then the need for these potential biases to be laid bare before the guideline audience, for them to examine carefully, assess, accept or reject, is compelling. The decision process in the absence of scientific evidence must be very explicit – and transparent – about the rationale, context and assumptions made at each stage. When evidence is lacking, recommendations are reflections of the professional opinions of those involved, comprised albeit of many elements.

Assumptions should not be made that one set of professional opinions, for example of those sitting as members of a guideline development group, represent or even accurately reflect the opinions of other members of the profession. Nor should it be assumed that those involved in recommendation development provide the professional opinions that must necessarily prevail, at least until scientific evidence is available.

But at least if the decision process is clear then professionals can use their professional judgement to make their own decisions about whether to follow the recommendation. The guideline users may or may not agree with these opinions and the recommendations derived from them. They may accept it or they may reject all or some of it. But they should be able to see the path that led to the final recommendation.

The role of opinion and context

There are several other stages in the process of deriving recommendations where subjectivity can be identified. Consideration of the evidence report which forms the basis of the guideline is unlikely to pass without comments from reviewers, even if reviewers are happy with its content, completeness, clinical relevance and so on. What is then to be done with these comments (an area that guideline developers have not yet resolved)? Should the comments be ignored, in which case the rationale for review is lost? But if comments are not ignored then a process of assessing and selecting comments must be undertaken – and this will inevitably be comprised of both objective and subjective elements.

The context in which the recommendations are intended to be followed will inevitably impinge on the derivation process. This influence of context can be seen in several ways. For example, the same evidence base and even the same evidence statements do not necessarily lead to the same recommendations being produced, a problem explored by Breen and Feder in Chapter 2. This difficulty is apparent when, for example, guidelines for a particular condition, or aspect of a condition, are produced in primary and in secondary care. Furthermore, although the same evidence base may be used, different recommendations can ensue. For example, despite using in essence the same evidence review, there were different recommendations in several areas in the guidelines for back pain of the American Agency for Health Care Policy and Research[6] and those led by the British Royal College of General Practitioners,[7] notably in areas such as surgical intervention. Contrasts such as these demonstrate how issues of professional, organisational and patient acceptability will be taken into consideration as will resource implications in the activity of turning evidence statements into evidence-linked guideline recommendations.

Recognition must be given to professional issues, no matter how undesirable it may be considered:[8]

establishing clinical guidelines is primarily a 'political' process in that it entails negotiating a common policy between conflicting interests. (p 243)

These interests may be the obvious political interests, but may also involve conflicting interests within and between different professional groups. What suits some professions in terms of recommended action may not suit others, no matter what the evidence says, and especially if the recommendations are perceived as threatening to professional autonomy, control or livelihood. Therefore, the need for clarity, explicitness and attribution is required when dealing with views in guideline development just as it is when dealing with scientific evidence.

In all these areas where subjectivity is a major component of the guideline development process, then it is likely that a process of consensus building will be required.

Consensus

There are a number of important considerations in the use of consensus methods in guideline development (*see also* Chapter 3):

- group membership
- agreement
- evidence presentation
- consensus building methods
- reaching consensus.

Group membership

The membership of the guideline development group is obviously a major determinant in the consensus process. It is their opinions, values, interpretation and use of evidence that shapes the final product. Careful choice of group membership could ensure consensus, as Skrabanek[2] has suggested:

The careful selection of participants guarantees a consensus. (p 1446)

Thus, selection criteria for group membership, and not just the identity of group members, should be clear and available for scrutiny, not least because bias in group membership could lead to bias in the shape of consensus.

Lomas[9] has identified three distinct types of consensus group membership (*see* Box 5.1). Despite the importance of panel group membership, few studies are yet available that examine the effect of panel composition on the process, although both Newton and colleagues[10] and Eccles and colleagues (Chapter 3) have undertaken an initial analysis.

Box 5.1: Three types of members of a consensus group

1 Clinical experts in the area being considered.
2 Experts in both the clinical and related aspects of the topic.
3 Non-expert or independent panel.

Criteria for inclusion in the panel centre on the degree of expertise that is required, which might be clinical, methodological, health economics or project management. Different areas and different requirements for the final guidelines should be used to help identify panel inclusion criteria. It must also be clear in what capacity the individuals are present on the panel. Are they there to use their expertise and voice their own opinions, or are they there representing a particular body, professional or otherwise? Thus, it should be clear who is on the panel, why they were included and whose views they represent. Any real or potential conflict of interest, or other vested interests, must also be made clear.

The problems associated with the bias of panels are sometimes difficult to deal with when the panel is uniprofessional and primarily concerned with intervention guidelines for a narrowly defined clinical procedure. When guidelines are developed by a multiprofessional group for disease management (e.g. in a complicated chronic disease such as type 2 diabetes or asthma) then, as expected, the problems are even more frequent and complex.

There can also be problems with inherent hierarchies amongst different professionals on the panel. The lack of knowledge input skills, roles and responsibilities that different professionals have in managing a complex disease add to the potential complications.

The process of developing consensus therefore is not only concerned with approaching agreement on content but also in ensuring that different professional perspectives are given due weight and attention.

The multiprofessional aspects of guideline development has important implications for consensus. Not least is the likelihood that the greater number and complexity of issues involved, and the professional issues brought by each individual to the group, will require more sophisticated consensus methods to be used, to enhance the likelihood of achieving consensus. Leape[4] and colleagues reported the results of a study of attempts to agree the indications for carotid endarterectomy. One group was a multiprofessional panel, the other was a uniprofessional panel comprising surgeons only. They found that, as they expected:

the AS [all surgical] panel found more indications for carotid endarterectomy appropriate and fewer inappropriate than did the multispeciality HSUS panel. (p 157)

The difficulties of reaching consensus are compounded when dealing with differing professional perspectives. This is an area where more formal, or structured, consensus methods may have an important role to play, for several reasons. The difficulties encountered when individuals dominate discussion can be tackled by using secret/confidential voting systems to gather views. Disagreement can then be dealt with by the consensus process and the chair, rather than the onus being left with individuals to resolve the issue. People have a framework in which to consider the issues rather than relying on personalities – it produces a formalised structural issue rather than a clash (perhaps one that cannot be resolved) of personalities and individuals. New, computerised, voting systems with instant feedback may offer a valuable addition to anonymous voting in consensus development.

Agreement

The degree to which the individual agrees with the other individuals involved and the degree to which the individual agrees with the point under consideration are two key elements of the process. We can assess the degree of agreement between individuals, and agreement with the point being considered, in a process which can be thought of as consensus measurement. We can also employ methods to bring about agreement where agreement either with each other or the issue is absent, which can be thought of as consensus development or consensus building. To measure the amount of agreement is easier than trying to bring about agreement when it is absent!

In a guideline development group some participants may agree with all that is being proposed, while others may only agree with certain elements of that proposed. Thus, not only must a distinction be drawn between the amount of agreement between participants, but there must also be distinction on the degree of agreement between participants on how much, and of which, elements are under consideration. For instance, all participants might agree with the general view being proposed but disagree on emphasis, on wording and so on. Therefore, there are several interrelated strands in the process involved in trying to produce a final view or version.

Approaches to agreement

The level of agreement that is considered necessary, or required, should be set out at the start of the guideline development process. For example, will a simple majority be acceptable, or must a certain proportion of group members be in agreement for consensus to be deemed to have been achieved? It should also be clear if these levels of agreement are applied for all aspects of process or if differential levels are to be used in different domains. For instance, a different level of agreement might be desirable for deciding on topics to be included in the scope of the guideline, in contrast to the level of agreement to be reached in disputes over particular wording of a recommendation. The exact mechanisms to be used will depend on several issues, such as the maturity of the group and the skills available to undertake consensus building. The actual development process being followed in terms of the guideline and its recommendations will also play a part.

Evidence presentation

The derivation of recommendations consists of the process of synthesising available evidence and combining with opinion. Thus, an important part of the process is receiving and then processing the available evidence. The way in which the available evidence is presented to members of the panel is both crucial and influential in the overall process of bringing evidence and opinion together. In trying to undertake this process, several approaches are feasible and desirable.

The presentation of information to the development group can be thought of as several stages. First, the evidence review is undertaken, then recommendations are drafted and, finally, revisions are made to recommendations. The evidence review should produce a document that presents the synthesised evidence in a clear, easy-to-follow format with evidence statements summarising key research findings (e.g. *see* the process described in Chapter 3). It should be made available to all group members before their discussions begin. After review of the evidence document, when accuracy, completeness, omissions and so on can be discussed, the initial draft of recommendations is undertaken. There are several approaches that can be used. For example, the project team, who often undertake the evidence review, might provide the first draft of recommendations that the guideline group can then discuss and reformulate. Alternatively, the guideline development group as a whole may try to formulate draft recommendations directly from the evidence statements.

In reality, most guidelines will employ a combination of both approaches. Where the evidence or professional opinion is quite clear about what the direction of the recommendation should be, and development group members are in agreement, then written drafts can be produced by one or two members of the project team before being brought back for final consideration by the guideline development group. The more difficult process of consensus building can then concentrate on areas where the evidence is equivocal or where disagreement between group members exists.

Consensus building methods

These are usually thought of as being in two broad types, formal (or structured) methods and informal (or unstructured). The most significant difference in approach is that structured methods usually employ an explicit, structured set of operating rules. Informal methods resemble more closely the decisions taken in groups, committees and other 'round table' discussion forums. Boundaries between formal and informal methods are not always clear, especially in their usage. A recent systematic review by Murphy and colleagues[11] of the use of consensus in guidelines provides greater detail about the various consensus building methods and an assessment of the scarce research in this field. They summarised the characteristics of informal and formal methods of consensus (*see* Table 5.1).

Principal methods of formal consensus development

Four main methods have been used in guideline development:

1 *Consensus development conferences.* Panel members meet together over a period of two days. They may hear presentations and receive written summaries of scientific evidence in a public forum. They then retire in private to produce consensus statements.[12] This method of consensus development conferences has been used more extensively in North America than in the UK.[13] Thompson and Kitson report their experience of the process in Chapter 4.

Table 5.1: Characteristics of consensus development methods (adapted from Murphy *et al.*, p. 3, table 1[11])

Consensus development method	Mailed questionnaires	Private decisions elicited	Formal feedback of group choices	Face-to-face contact	Interaction structured	Aggregation method
Informal	No	No	No	Yes	No	Implicit
Consensus development conference	No	No	No	Yes	No	Implicit
Delphi method	Yes	Yes	Yes	No	Yes	Explicit
Nominal group technique	No	Yes	Yes	Yes	Yes	Explicit
RAND appropriateness method	Yes	Yes	Yes	Yes	Yes	Explicit

2 *Delphi method*. Members independently assess and vote on the importance of the issues presented to them. Panel members do not meet face to face, thus it is primarily conducted as a series of voting rounds conducted by post. Voting rounds are repeated until consensus ensues or until no further convergence occurs.[14]

3 *Nominal group technique*. Expert panels are facilitated by either a topic expert or someone who is not a clinical expert but has credibility with the panel. The method entails going round the panel and collecting ideas from each member in a rigorous and structured process. These ideas are then discussed, clarified and ranked. The final ranking is the consensus reached by the panel.[15]

4 *RAND appropriateness method*. This is increasingly being used and combines elements of other methods. It has been broadly defined as:[3]

a structured group judgement method for incorporating expert clinical judgement with the scientific literature in assessing medical procedures. (p 1)

It is a technique that incorporates various elements of different consensus approaches including face-to-face meetings, voting, use of structured reviews of scientific evidence. This method has been used in the US in helping to develop clinical guidelines about, for example, low back pain.[3]

The RAND method is also currently being used in the UK to develop review criteria for type 2 diabetes, asthma and angina. Whilst this approach seems to be a valuable way of combining scientific literature and expert opinion it is likely that its use in guideline development will still be a long way short of providing an 'objective, value free, scientific' method for producing consensus in guideline development. As with other consensus methods, a recommendation will still have to be drafted, discussed and voted upon. Thus, subjective elements will still compose a major component of this relatively structured approach. Nevertheless, one of the features of the RAND appropriateness method approach is that it is very structured, well documented and explicit and these characteristics alone may make it more preferable to most of the other methods currently used.

Reaching consensus

To vote word-by-word on the wording of a recommendation using a structured consensus method would potentially be a time-consuming and ultimately overcomplicated means of agreeing a recommendation, especially one where the general direction of the recommendation is agreed by all. Indeed, if the development group are all agreed with the general direction of a recommendation, but the actual wording is causing disagreement, then an informal consensus process might suffice. An explicit and prior agreed level of assent could be used and discussion could be followed by, for example, a simple vote – perhaps a showing of hands.

However, if there is considerable disagreement between individuals and with the general direction of the recommendation, especially if it is considered a key recommendation or is thought to be a controversial area, then a more structured approach may be worthwhile and necessary to achieve agreement, explicitness and credibility.

This bringing together of the various views to reach the consensus presented can be quite simple and relatively unstructured (such as a simple majority vote), or much more sophisticated and structured using methods such as multiple round voting. The more sophisticated and structured approaches tend to be the more explicit.

The use of consensus in guidelines

There is a view that if rigorous scientific evidence is not available, recommendations should not be made. Such views include concerns over recommending a course of action for which there is no supporting or contrary evidence, and which may later turn out to be harmful to patients. In such instances practitioners are then left to their own devices in terms of decision making. However, this lack of direction is not always useful for practitioners who have turned to the guidelines, presumably looking for direction.

Woolf and colleagues[1] describe the problem faced by the United States Preventive Services Task Force when some recommendations were given a C-level grading, which was defined as:

There is insufficient evidence to make a recommendation for or against consideration in the periodic health examination. (p 523)

This neutral stance presented problems:[1]

the most obvious being that many clinicians found it unhelpful, giving no guidance in either direction. The scientific dogmatism seemed out of place with the rest of medicine; much of what is done in clinical practice has not yet been proven to improve health outcomes. (p 527)

In terms of clinical guidelines there is an ongoing debate about the role consensus, and in particular consensus-based recommendations and guidelines, should have. As Lomas[9] puts it:

Is the purpose of recommendations from consensus processes to establish the best possible guidance for clinical care despite imperfect or incomplete evidence, or is it to promulgate science based only on watertight conclusions derived from methodologically incontestable studies. (p 52)

Even if the second view is the preferred option, a process of consensus will still be undertaken to arrive at recommendations and guidelines based on methodologically sound studies. There is a role for consensus in guidelines even if they only consider scientific literature and decide only to make recommendations in areas where there is scientific evidence to support them. This is for several reasons, not least the subjective process of turning research findings into recommendations that clinicians can relate to and follow in their everyday practice. For example, Kanouse and colleagues have argued:[16]

The consensus panel is supposed to translate biomedical research findings into clinically meaningful recommendations. To do its job well, the panel should be well informed about both the current state of science and the current state of practice. (p 242)

The application of consensus methods in guidelines development lies:[17]

where unanimity of opinion does not exist owing to lack of scientific evidence or where there is contradictory evidence on an issue. (p 376–7)

Science is not value-free, we all know that. But scientific method should be as explicit and as open to scrutiny as possible to allow the value judgements taken to be seen in the light of our own values and judgements.

Reproducibility

A major issue for guidelines development and for the consensus process used is that of reproducibility. It is argued that the development process should be such that another group, given the same remit, scientific information and methods, should reach essentially the same conclusions and hence recommendations.[18] However, given the considerable resources involved in guideline development, this has not been empirically tested on complete national guidelines.

There is some information available about this issue from a study by Pearson and colleagues.[19] They used three groups to develop algorithms for two conditions: the management of dyspepsia and the management of sinusitis. The basic process for each condition involved presenting the panels with a selection of literature and a seed algorithm, produced by the project team. The panels, using elements of a nominal group process and a modified Delphi technique, produced their final versions of the algorithms. Finding that there was a reasonable degree of similarity in the dyspepsia algorithms but less agreement for the algorithm concerned with sinusitis, they concluded that:[19]

It seems likely that the more detailed and literature supported the seed algorithm is, the more reproducible the final group consensus will be. (p 652)

Attributes of the consensus process in guideline development

In guideline development, where the opportunities for disagreement, interpretation and competing views are great because scientific evidence does not provide the reference frame for discussion, there is always a need for clear, well-structured and visible development process to be in place. The basic principles of project management and their application are indispensable.

In an evidence-based guideline, we would expect a clear account of the methods used, including the methods of assessing and synthesising evidence, to be made available in the final guideline report. This would include a clear explanation of the rules of evidence grading and the rules used to derive and link evidence statements with the resultant recommendations. This is required to allow the user to assess whether the guideline possesses the attributes that we expect of evidence-based guidelines, namely, validity, reproducibility, reliability and credibility.[20] The appraisal instruments that are available are one way of trying to ensure that the necessary requirements of a robust process to develop evidence-based guidelines are met (*see* Cluzeau and Littlejohns, Chapter 6).

Ideally the same rigour, transparency and reporting methods that are applied to the process of assessing and dealing with bias in producing the evidence base from published literature should be applied to the process of using consensus in guideline development.

In terms of consensus guidelines, Lomas[9] has argued that clear information, criteria and methods for the following should be available (*see* Box 5.2).

Box 5.2: Consensus guidelines

1 topic selected
2 membership of the consensus group
3 nature and extent of background preparation
4 inclusion/exclusion criteria for information inputs
5 type of group processes and definition of consensus
6 criteria for qualification as a recommendation
7 preparation process and format of report

Given that in reality most national guidelines will for the foreseeable future consist of recommendations that combine evidence (to differing degrees) with opinion (elicited through a consensus process of some kind), the processes used to develop the guideline, review evidence and build consensus should all be transparent and available for examination. The user expects to be able to clearly follow the guideline, clearly distinguish evidence statements from recommendations and to identify the linkages that have been made between the evidence, summarised evidence statements and recommendations. The process between these elements should be available and clear to the guideline user.

Conclusion

The view expressed by Woolf and colleagues,[1] that:

A fundamental lesson learned by the USPSTF [United States Preventative Services Task Force] is the need for a policy on making recommendations when there is insufficient evidence. (p 534)

is one that guideline developers should address, and reach conclusions about as soon as possible. For guideline development will always involve subjectivity somewhere in the process. If this is unacceptable to individuals, and groups, then it is unlikely that they will be happy with guideline development.

Although some argue that no recommendation should be produced if there is no scientific evidence to support the action proposed, many consider that this will always leave vast areas of clinical practice without guidance about what is currently considered appropriate action, professionals will continue to hold and voice opinions. Whether they are based on evidence or not, if actions are being suggested in the absence of firm scientific evidence this should be clearly visible, so allowing professionals to exercise their clinical and professional judgement in deciding whether they follow that recommended action or not.

Decisions about clinical practice will always be a mixture of evidence-based actions and opinion-led actions. What they should all have in common, however, is that they are actions that can be explained and understood, and the rationale underlying them made visible. The move towards making decisions underlying actions explicit is one that should be welcomed and followed. The challenge, then, is for professionals to continue to bring to bear their professional judgement on difficult issues and enable scrutiny of the explicit processes by which that judgement was exercised and decisions reached. There is no doubt that many professional opinions on best practice that once prevailed have been shown to be wrong as evidence is assembled that disproves those opinions. Are we absolutely sure that this never happens with evidence?

References

1 Woolf S, DiGuiseppi CG, Atkins D and Kamerow DB (1996) Developing evidence-based clinical practice guidelines: lessons learned by the US Preventive Services Task Force. *Annual Review of Public Health*, **17**: 511–38.

2 Skrabanek P (1990) Nonsensus consensus. *Lancet*, **335**: 1446–7.

3 Shekelle PG and Schriger DL (1993) *Using the Appropriateness Method in Clinical Practice Guideline Development*. RAND, Santa Monica, CA.

4 Leape L, Park RE, Kahan JP and Brook RH (1992) Group judgements of appropriateness: the effect of panel composition. *Quality Assurance in Health Care*, **4**: 151–9.

5 Fletcher JW and Woolf SH (1994) Royal HD Consensus development for producing diagnostic procedure guidelines: SPECT brain perfusion imaging with exametazine. *Journal of Nuclear Medicine*, **35**: 2003–10.

6 Agency for Health Care Policy and Research (1994) *Management Guidelines for Acute Low Back Pain*. AHCPR/US Department of Health and Human Services, Rockville, MD.

7 Waddell G, Feder G, McIntosh A, Lewis M and Hutchinson A (1996) *Low Back Pain Evidence Review*. Royal College of General Practitioners, London.

8 Armstrong D, Tatford P, Fry J and Armstrong P (1992) Development of clinical guidelines in a health district: an attempt to find consensus. *Quality in Health Care*, **1**: 241–4.

9   Lomas J (1991) Words without action? The production, dissemination and impact of consensus recommendations. *Annual Review of Public Health*, **12**: 41–65.

10 Newton J, Hutchinson A, Steen N *et al.* (1992) Educational potential of medical audit: observations from a study of small groups setting standards. *Quality in Health Care*, **1**: 256–9.

11 Murphy MK *et al.* (1998) Consensus development methods, and their use in clinical guideline development. *Health Technology Assessment*, **2**(3).

12 Fink A, Kosecoff J, Chassin M and Brook RH (1984) Consensus methods: characteristics and guidelines for use. *American Journal of Public Health*, **74**: 979–83.

13 Kosecoff J, Kanouse DE, Rogers WH, McCloskey L, Winslow CM and Brook RH (1987) Effects of the National Institutes of Health consensus development program on physician practice. *JAMA*, **258**: 2708–13.

14 Dalkey NC and Helmer O (1963) An experimental application of the Delphi method to the use of experts. *Management Science*, **9**: 458–67.

15 Delbecq A and Van de Ven A (1971) A group process model for problem identification and program planning. *Journal of Applied Behavioral Science*, **7**: 467–92.

16 Kanouse DE, Brook RH, Winkler JD, Kosecoff J, Berry SH *et al.* (1989) *Changing Medical Practice through Technology Assessment: An Evaluation of the NIH Consensus Development Program*. Health Administration Press, Ann Arbor, MI.

17 Jones J and Hunter D (1995) Consensus methods for medical and health services research. *BMJ*, **311**: 376–80.

18 Grimshaw J and Russell I (1993) Developing health gain through clinical guidelines: I. Developing scientifically valid guidelines. *Quality in Health Care*, **2**: 243–8.

19 Pearson SD, Margolis CZ, Davis S, Schrieber LK, Sokol N and Gottlieb LK (1995) Is consensus reproducible? A study of an algorithmic guidelines development process. *Medical Care*, **33**: 643–60.

20 Field M and Lohr KN (eds) (1992) *Guidelines for Clinical Practice: From Development to Use*. Institute of Medicine/National Academy Press, Washington DC.

6
Assessing the quality of guidelines

Françoise Cluzeau and Peter Littlejohns

Guideline users repeatedly seek guidance on the provenance of both local and national guidelines. Research referred to in this chapter supports the often expressed user view that there are often conflicting recommendations offered by development groups, usually from the same evidence base. One method of combating this problem is to develop systems for appraising the quality of guidelines. This can help developers and users alike, by contributing to a common standard. Here the authors describe international approaches to guideline appraisal and discuss the introduction of a new appraisal programme for the National Health Service.

Introduction

It is disconcerting to find, in the current guidelines, so many unsubstantiated, inaccurate and occasionally frankly incorrect statements. Inexact science is both aesthetically distasteful and intrinsically debilitating. Moreover, many physicians will look no further than these publications if hypertension is not their speciality – indeed the guidelines are specifically addressed to such persons. Thus misconceptions and inapt procedures risk perpetuation. Especially unfortunate is the general avoidance in these reports of discussion of important current controversies. Thus in some respects the publications show more affinity with the theological orthodoxy demanded in earlier centuries than with contemporary scientific debate. (Robertson, 1994[1])

Thus four national guidelines on hypertension (American,[2] British,[3] Canadian,[4] New Zealand[5]) and one international guideline sponsored by the World Health Organisation (WHO)[6] on the management of raised blood pressure are dismissed by Ian Robertson.[1] Like many other commentators, he is concerned that eminent experts, reviewing virtually the same literature can come up with differing recommendations. This finding is even more intriguing when it is known that some individuals were on more than one committee. Nor are these merely semantic differences, interesting only to the methodological ruminators. When these guidelines were applied to real patients in a general practice population in the UK only about a third of patients met the treatment criteria of all four guidelines.[7] If the New Zealand guidelines were taken as a standard, which had calculated absolute risks for a cardiovascular event, half of the patients with uncontrolled hypertension by the US criteria would be treated unnecessarily and 31% of those classified as having controlled hypertension by the Canadian guidelines would be denied beneficial treatment.

Similar variations were recently reported by Thomson and colleagues in a comparison of British guidelines on anticoagulant treatment in atrial fibrillation.[8] They found that guidelines varied considerably in their advice for anticoagulant treatment to the extent that, if applied to patients they could potentially have a significant effect on outcomes. The authors also suggested that these differences would have important implications for the use of anticoagulant services.

Many reasons have been put forward to explain this variability (see Box 6.1). They range from methodological issues relating to the presentation of risk[9] to possible bias introduced through conflicts of

---

Box 6.1: Possible reasons for variation in guidelines recommendations

- Lack of evidence
  (no research, research not found, poor research).

- Differing interpretation of evidence
  (difficulties in agreeing on quality of research, difficulites in extrapolating research findings to clinical situation).

- Different values given to anticipated outcome
  (perception of risk,[9] importance of cost[10]).

- Dubious achievement of consensus.

interest.[10,11] The usefulness of guidelines in improving the quality of patient care will depend on how these issues are addressed and how realistic conclusions can be reached. The 'guideline sceptics' argue that the difficulties are likely to be insurmountable;[12,13] the advocates suggest that it is too early to say, as our understanding of guideline development and implementation is still embryonic.[14]

This chapter will adopt a stance closer to the latter. We will argue that a key first step is to develop the ability to assess the quality of guidelines with reliable and valid criteria. Such criteria will allow us to explore and understand the reasons behind guideline variability. Of course, the creation of the recommendations is an important but only first step in the guideline process. If guidelines are to improve patient care, the difficulties of dissemination and implementation[15] also have to be overcome. There remains debate about how narrowly or broadly quality is defined in the context of guideline creation, and who holds responsibility. The determinants of success at each stage (i.e. development, implementation and dissemination), are not necessarily compatible. For example, evidence-based national guidelines produced by experts are more likely to be valid but least likely to be implemented.[16] Local guidelines where there is user involvement in their creation will increase the likelihood of their use, but not their validity.[17]

This chapter describes the initial stages of a research programme designed to provide a practical approach to the appraisal of clinical guidelines and explores the issues involved using the results of a recent appraisal.

How do you assess the quality of guidelines?

Background

In the early 1990s, it was becoming increasingly apparent that the guideline industry initiated in the US was beginning to emerge in the UK.[18] There was increasing concern that duplication should be avoided and benefit maximised through some process of co-ordination.[19] In June 1993, the National Health Service Executive convened a national workshop to explore these issues and identify how to marry the validity of centralised guideline creation with the local ownership needed to ensure their implementation. An important conclusion of the day's deliberations was the need to create a mechanism to appraise guidelines critically, in the same way that research literature was being systematically assessed by the Cochrane Collaboration. In seeking how this should be undertaken, more questions were raised than solutions proffered. For example – What criteria should be used to assess guidelines? Whose perspective should you take? Who should do the appraisal?

It was decided that further research and development was required. A joint working group was set up between the Health Care Evaluation Unit at St. George's Medical School, the Health Services Research Unit from Aberdeen University and the Royal College of Physicians. The aim was to produce a generic instrument to appraise guidelines in relation to their wider application within the NHS. The instrument should be capable of being applied by anyone (clinician, purchaser and researcher) interested in the guideline. There was general acknowledgement at this early stage that this was going to be a complex task, and that the instrument would need extensive testing and reviewing before it could be widely adopted.

Experience in the US had already demonstrated the inherent difficulties in producing such an appraisal instrument.[20] The process commenced by reviewing the existing criteria developed by the Institute of Medicine (IoM) [21] and the McMaster group.[22] Ideally, information on the ability of guidelines to bring about the anticipated health outcomes when they are followed should be available. Criteria would then be derived from the identification of the determinants of a successful outcome.[23] In reality there is a virtual absence of this type of evaluative information for most guidelines. In recognition of this, both institutions concluded that appraisal criteria would have to be based on the *rigour of the development process and the face validity of the guidelines.*

The criteria assessed whether developers overcame the many potential biases during guideline development and emphasised the importance of identifying scientific evidence and using appropriate group consensus techniques. Despite this common conceptual approach, there were differences between the two sets of criteria. While the McMaster criteria were tailored for appraisal of guidelines by individual clinicians or local users, the IoM criteria were more detailed and inclusive of all the dimensions against which guidelines would be appraised in future. Thus, the IoM provisional instrument was identified as the most suitable for use in a pilot study. The structure of the IoM instrument also provided a more evaluative framework for making a judgement about the development process and face validity of guidelines.

The pilot study

The Institute of Medicine identifies eight desirable attributes for clinical guidelines. The original appraisal instrument contains 46 questions divided into eight sections, each corresponding to an attribute, apart from *documentation* which is addressed through the other attributes. The questions ask whether information is available on the development process and about the quality of that information. Many of the sections in the IoM instrument were considered to be inappropriate for current guideline development activity in the UK. Therefore, some questions were excluded. The revised version contained a total of 37 questions. Some of the questions were also reworded to make them more applicable to UK practice. The questions called for five categories of answers, for example, 'Is there a description of the population to which the guidelines are meant to apply?' answer: (*a*) 'yes' and satisfactory quality, (*b*) 'yes' and conditionally or unsatisfactory quality, (*c*) 'no' and unimportant or minor omission, (*d*) 'no' and major omission, (*e*) 'can't tell/don't know/not applicable'. Each section was preceded by a description of the attribute.

Five UK guidelines were selected to test these criteria. The rationale for selecting the guidelines was whether there was documented evidence on their development, or evidence of their application. Attempts were also made at including both nationally recognised guidelines, or guidelines endorsed by professional organisations, and those produced by local physicians for local use. Available background information on the development of the guidelines was collected. This included peer-reviewed papers, background articles on which the evidence for the recommendations was based, and other documentation. Lead people in the production of guidelines were contacted for more detailed information although this proved difficult as in some cases no one individual would take responsibility.

Seven individuals with experience or an interest in clinical guidelines appraised the guidelines. They comprised: two purchasers, one hospital clinician, one nurse, one general practitioner and two public health physicians. Each was issued with the five sets of guidelines and the accompanying documentation and explanatory information about the instrument. They were also asked to provide comments on the format of the instrument. The assessments were done independently.

Results of the pilot study

The details of the pilot study have been published elsewhere.[24] In summary, most guidelines performed well on clarity of content and on the composition of the development group. All provided a description of the patients likely to be affected by the recommendations, although the quality of the description was judged to be deficient in three of the guidelines. Patients' preferences were thought to have been overlooked in the majority of cases but the omission was not always considered to be major. Only two guidelines gave an indication that they might have been externally reviewed before publication. All guidelines performed poorly against validity criteria, including the collection and assessment of evidence, references, consensus methods and expected health outcomes. Qualitative descriptions on health benefits and risks were thought to have been provided in some cases, but quantitative information, and economic costs associated with the application of guidelines were lacking overall. All guidelines failed to indicate when they would be updated or reviewed.

Conclusions from the pilot study

A number of issues emerged from the pilot study. First, it was clear that there was insufficient information on the development process of the appraised guidelines, in particular about the type of evidence used, methods of consensus, health outcomes, cost-effectiveness and resource implications. Most of the Institute of Medicine criteria asked for information expected to be found in a detailed background document, but none of the guidelines had such a document. It has been suggested that synthesised information of the development process in the form of structured abstracts provides essential information needed to assess the validity and applicability of guidelines.[25] Certainly, the guidelines which performed best in the pilot study also had more detailed background documentation, emphasising the importance of such evidence for independent review.[26] The lack of information is more likely to induce value judgements. Appraisers in the pilot reported that on several occasions their responses had been based on their personal knowledge of guidelines rather than on available information.

The second issue raised in the pilot was that the IoM criteria may have represented a 'gold standard' which would be unlikely to be achieved in most circumstances. Prospective assessment of outcomes, and estimates of risks and benefits associated with different types of management are often inaccurate.[27] Research-based evidence is lacking in most disease areas and even the best researched subjects are often based on patchy evidence. When there is strong evidence, for instance from large randomised clinical trials, it may be difficult to translate these into recommendations, because there are often important differences between the selected study population and the patients seen in clinical practice,[28] or because the results only apply to a subgroup of the population and therefore cannot be extrapolated to the general patient population.[13] Since studies cannot predict with certainty the outcome for an individual it is likely that most guidelines will be 'hybrid' documents combining a mixture of evidence and consensus.[28,29] Thus, evidence of how consensus is reached and the participants involved is of interest for gauging the likely validity of guidelines.

A third issue raised in the pilot study was how to form a global assessment of the guidelines on the basis of their performance against individual criteria. For example, should there be a minimum number of 'mandatory' criteria, or requirements for guidelines to be recommended?[30] A possible approach would be to devise a scoring system to measure the performance of guidelines against the criteria. This is technically complex as guidelines vary enormously in terms of the topics they cover, type of management, interventions, diagnosis, and the purpose for which they have been produced. Therefore, it is important to design a scoring system that takes into account the nature of the condition or topic covered by the guidelines.

Establishing the reliability of the criteria is technically complex. This is partly due to the multidimensional nature of guidelines and partly to the subjective nature of the appraisal process. Making the criteria more explicit minimises the need for inference and therefore is likely to increase agreement between reviewers.[31] However, there may be systematic differences of opinion between professional groups. For example, Leape and colleagues observed differences between surgical and multidisciplinary panels on appropriateness of indications for carotid endarterectomy, the surgical panel being more likely to favour operative treatment than the multispeciality panel.[32] Similar results were found by Scott and Black[33] in a study comparing ratings of appropriateness of cholecystectomy by a mixed panel and an all surgical panel. Areas of disagreement between reviewers can be addressed through nominal group consensus.[34] This technique is reliant on the group leader whose expertise in co-ordinating groups is accepted by all health professionals.

The reviewers in the pilot study were from different professional backgrounds but were not expected to represent their professional groups. While the ratings were similar across the professions, the comments made by the reviewers provide some insight into differences of perspective that may exist between professional groups. For example, the need for patient education and patient involvement in developing the guidelines was mentioned more often by the nurse than by her medical colleagues. It is likely that judgement is influenced by personal experience of the work in the particular clinical area.[35] Differences of perception between professions obviously need to be recognised in the selection of reviewers for appraisal of guidelines.

Finally, the IoM instrument deals exclusively with the development of the guidelines. It was thought that the dissemination, implementation and long-term impact on practice and patient outcome needed to be assessed in parallel to the development process as they are inherent to the effectiveness of guidelines.[15] It was proposed that the instrument should include a section specifying the context in which the guidelines will be applied, on local protocol development, dissemination and implementation. Other suggestions called for a section on clinical audit and the mechanisms for monitoring the performance of the guidelines for reporting the results to guideline users. Appraisers' comments on the format of the instrument varied from 'intelligible and comprehensive' to 'rather long and off-putting'. It was suggested that the content of the questionnaire could be made clearer by using categorical questions that would call for a 'Yes' or 'No' answer.

A new appraisal instrument

On the basis of the pilot study a revised instrument was developed[36] and a research project designed to test its reliability and validity. This was to include a national survey of guidelines in a number of disease areas. A research protocol was successfully submitted to the national Research and Development (R&D) initiative by the Health Care Evaluation Unit in collaboration with the Health Services Research Unit, Aberdeen University and the Department of Primary Care St. Bartholomew's Hospital Medical School.

Implicit in the revised appraisal instrument was the notion that clinical guidelines are 'systematically developed statements to assist practitioner and patient decisions about appropriate healthcare for specific clinical circumstances'.[21] They are an attempt to distil a large body of medical knowledge into a convenient format and contain explicit recommendations to inform clinicians.[25] Thus, the appraisal framework must contain criteria that will address both the scientific validity of the guidelines and the operational factors involved in their application.

The purpose of the instrument is twofold. First, it aims to provide a structured framework for appraising the validity and content of existing guidelines, using a set of reliable criteria. Secondly, it aims to encourage the systematic development of new guidelines and to be used as a checklist or *aide-mémoire* by guideline developers.

Structure and content of the new appraisal instrument

The instrument has 37 questions divided into three dimensions corresponding to the IoM attributes (*see* Appendix). Since the instrument assesses the rigour of the development process of the guidelines, it relies heavily on the quality of background documentation.

Questions ask whether information is available on different components of the development process and require judgement about the quality of the information. Responses to each question are typically 'yes' or 'no'. There are two categories 'not sure' and 'not applicable' to accommodate cases where appraisers may feel unsure or the criterion is not relevant to the guidelines.

Dimension I. Rigour of development process

This contains 20 questions and is designed to reflect the attributes of guideline validity and reproducibility. It assesses the following:

(*a*) *Responsibility for guideline development.* The responsibility for the development of the guidelines, external funding or support that might have been received and the potential biases that could have occurred should be clearly identified. Sponsors are likely to have different priorities.[37] For example, a Royal College may be concerned with maintaining its members' knowledge and expertise. A government-funded body, on the other hand, may be primarily interested in ensuring that healthcare expenditure does not exceed the budget. These separate interests may lead to differences between recommendations for guidelines covering the same topic.

(b) *Development group.* The composition of the group involved in the development of guidelines has a considerable impact on their validity and acceptability. Since the management of most conditions is shared by a range of clinicians, it is important that these groups be represented at some stage of the development process and potential disagreements between stakeholders need to be resolved in order to ensure a sense of ownership and perceived value.[38] Obviously, the composition of the group will vary depending on the topic covered by the guidelines. Guideline developers should ensure that the group includes representatives from interested parties whose views will be considered in the formulation of the final recommendations.

(c) *Selection, interpretation and assessment of evidence.* Evidence-based guideline development requires explicit linkage between recommendations and the quality of the supporting evidence. This involves three stages: first the selection of evidence including the strategy for the literature search, bibliographic databases used, sources of information and exclusion criteria. This allows the incorporation of relevant studies on specific patient populations from a relatively unbiased position. The second component is the interpretation and grading of evidence (*see* Chapters 2 and 3). Thirdly, the results of the synthesis should be clearly reported. This transparent process should help demonstrate that there is a direct relationship between the final recommendations and the underlying evidence.[39]

Systematic reviews should be the preferred option when there is a solid body of research. However, such research in many clinical areas either does not exist or is inadequate. In the absence of rigorous studies it should be possible to use expert opinion to develop guidelines, provided the methods for reaching consensus, the strength of consensus and areas of uncertainty or discordance are explicitly reported[40] (*see also* Chapter 5). Several consensus methods have been used, including the Delphi and Glazer techniques, although their relative usefulness has been questioned.[41]

(d) *Formulation of recommendations.* Since deriving recommendations from the evidence is one of the most important aspects of guideline development and also one of the most complex, guideline authors should keep a detailed record of the methods used to derive the recommendations. This record could be presented as a flowchart or 'map', showing for each recommendation the stages and type of evidence used (e.g. randomised control trials, expert opinion in the absence of strong evidence). This explicit approach enables the user to make an informed judgement about the rationale and methods under-pinning the final recommendations.[42]

(e) *Peer review and updating.* Peer review and piloting can help test the applicability and relevance of the guidelines to the local setting and identify practical problems that can be rectified prior to the publication of the guidelines. Evidence-based guidelines also need regular updating to incorporate new research findings. Therefore, details on expiry date should be given, and the methods that will be used for updating them.

Dimension 2. Context and content

This dimension contains 12 items and addresses the attributes of guideline reliability, applicability, flexibility and clarity.

(a) *Aims and objectives of the guidelines.* In developing a guideline, the developers should formulate a number of questions to be answered. For example, a guideline may be written to clarify or resolve controversies, or to encourage more effective practice. A number of criteria have been suggested to appraise the relative importance of topics selected for guideline development, including: the prevalence of a condition or frequency of a procedure, economic costs of the condition and intervention.[43] As with any research methodology, the initial questions should be precise. The development group should be explicit in defining the outcomes.[44]

(b) *Presentation of recommendations, exceptions and patients' preferences.* This refers to the target population, the circumstances under which the guidelines apply and the clarity of the recommendations. Information should be given about the patients that are meant to be covered and exceptions for using the guidelines. For example, the guidelines should include details such as age range, and clinical description. Some statement should also be made about how patient preferences might be taken into account in applying the recommendations. It is increas-ingly recognised that patients have an important role to play in clinical decision making and that their experiences need to be recognised alongside scientific forms of evidence.[45] Definitions of terms should be clear, language unambiguous, and final recommendations presented in a format that can be easily assimilated by busy clinicians. For example, the use of prompts in consultation with patients has been associated with changes in clinicians' behaviour.[46,47]

(c) *Likely costs and benefits.* The issue of the likely costs associated with the recommended treatment is often overlooked in guideline development. Yet if guidelines are to play a part in promoting cost-effective care they must include some indication of the costs that might be incurred from the proposed management and weigh them against the potential health benefits. Thus, it is important that the cost component be dealt with during the development of the guidelines. Guideline authors need to provide details of the methods used to calculate prospective costs and benefits and assumptions made.

Dimension 3. Application of guidelines

This contains five questions addressing the implementation, dissemination and monitoring strategies.

(a) *Dissemination and implementation strategy.* The successful introduction of guidelines is reliant on the adoption of dissemination and implementation strategies that take into consideration a complex web of behavioural and contextual factors. These aspects should be addressed at the development stages. For instance, nationally produced guidelines may need to be adapted for local use to reflect detailed operational issues and precise organisational arrangements. It is likely that dissemination and implementation strategies will have to be tailored to the context in which guidelines will be used.[46]

(b) *Monitoring.* Evaluating and monitoring the uptake and impact of guidelines are important components. Some indication should be given about the audit criteria that might be used to judge whether the recommended standards are achieved.[23] These could include routine collection of data on patients' outcomes.

The user guide

Earlier in this chapter we noted that making the appraisal criteria as explicit as possible reduces the need for inference. To ensure that the questions in the new appraisal instrument are interpreted consistently a user guide has been designed that contains detailed explanation for each question. Its aim is to assist users of the instrument by clarifying potentially ambiguous terms and by providing examples of circumstances when a 'Yes' answer may be appropriate. Because the appraisal instrument is generic and therefore designed to be applied to a wide range of guidelines it would be impossible for the user guide to cover all possible circumstances in which a 'Yes' or 'No' may be given. Instead, it is intended to help appraisers make an informed judgement by reducing uncertainties and assumptions that they may otherwise have to make.

The main study

A national survey was first conducted to identify guidelines that had been produced between 1991 an 1996 on coronary disease (CHD), asthma, breast cancer, lung cancer and depression. Altogether, 472 guidelines were identified. The details of the survey have been published elsewhere.[48] A total of 60 guidelines (15 per disease group) was then selected from the database for appraisal. Lung cancer guidelines were excluded because only 12 had been identified in the survey. All 12 national guidelines were selected and 48 local guidelines were drawn through a random sample. As we noted earlier, detailed documentation is important for appraising the quality of guidelines. Therefore, guideline authors were asked to provide information describing how their guidelines had been developed with the help of a questionnaire – 53 out of 60 responded. Each guideline was assessed by six appraisers from different professional backgrounds. In this chapter we present a description of how well the guidelines performed against a selection of questions in the appraisal instrument (*see* Tables 6.1 and 6.2). The performance of each guideline against the criteria is described by using the most frequent response of the six appraisers. A guideline was judged to have met a criterion if at least four out of the six appraisers had given a 'Yes' answer.

The body responsible for developing or endorsing the guidelines had been clearly defined in 58 (96%) guidelines. Although most guidelines (53) had provided a description of their development group, only nine (15%) were thought to have had representatives of all key disciplines. The development group was more likely to be representative if guidelines had been produced after 1993 ($\chi^2 = 5.84$, $p < 0.05$). Sources of evidence used for the recommendations had been reported in over half the guidelines (38, 60%), but the search for evidence was judged to be comprehensive for only nine (15%) of guidelines. Four (7%) guidelines had provided adequate assessment of evidence. Locally produced guidelines were less likely to have been based on a comprehensive search of information ($\chi^2 = 36.5$, $p < 0.001$) and assessment of evidence ($\chi^2 = 38.7$, $p < 0.001$) than their national counterparts. Methods used for formulating the recommendations (i.e. consensus methods) were adequate for nine (15%) guidelines and five (8%) guidelines were thought to have explicit links between evidence and recommendations. These links were more likely to be explicit in the national guidelines (χ^2 = 37.4, $p < 0.001$) and in those produced after 1993 (χ^2 = 6.4, $p < 0.05$). Most asthma guidelines referred to the British Thoracic Society guidelines, although only one specifically identified where their recommendations differed, and most depression guidelines mentioned the 1992 consensus statement.

Conclusion

In this chapter we have described the main characteristics of a new appraisal instrument and have presented the initial results of its application to a sample of UK clinical guidelines. Developing reliable criteria is a complex process which involves extensive testing and reviewing and is conceptually similar to the development of measurement instruments such as the Overview Quality Assessment Questionnaire for evaluating the scientific quality of research reviews.[49] This includes validity and reliability testing.[50] Initial analyses from the main study suggest that the appraisal instrument is reliable and valid. However, work is in progress to identify those criteria which are most predictive in assessing evidence-based guidelines. For example, a distinction may need to be made between the criteria addressing

Table 6.1: Frequency of responses for each question by type of development of guidelines (percentage of valid responses)

Type of guidelines:	National		Local		
Number of guidelines:	13		47		
Maximum number of responses:	78		282		
	Yes	No[a]	Yes	No[a]	χ^2
Question 6	68 (88)	9 (12)	229 (81)	52 (19)	2.0 $p > 0.05$
Question 7	30 (39)	47 (61)	77 (27)	204 (73)	3.9 $p < 0.05$
Question 8	59 (78)	17 (22)	170 (60)	111 (40)	7.6 $p < 0.001$
Question 9	42 (55)	34 (45)	57 (20)	224 (80)	36.5 $p < 0.001$
Question 11	30 (39)	47 (61)	27 (10)	253 (90)	38.7 $p < 0.001$
Question 13	43 (56)	34 (44)	51 (18)	230 (82)	44.4 $p < 0.001$
Question 15	33 (43)	44 (57)	34 (12)	246 (88)	37.4 $p < 0.001$

[a] Includes 'Not sure' and 'Not applicable' responses.

Table 6.2: Frequency of responses for each question by year of development of guidelines (percentage of valid responses)

Year of development:	1992–93		1994–95		
Number of guidelines:	14		38		
Maximum number of responses:	84		228		
	Yes	No[a]	Yes	No[a]	χ^2
Question 6	78 (94)	5 (6)	189 (83)	38 (17)	5.8 $p<0.05$
Question 7	17 (20)	66 (80)	85 (37)	142 (63)	7.9 $p<0.05$
Question 8	61 (74)	21 (26)	151 (66)	76 (33)	1.7 $p>0.05$
Question 9	23 (28)	59 (72)	68 (74)	159 (70)	0.1 $p>0.05$
Question 11	10 (12)	71 (88)	44 (19)	184 (81)	2.0 $p>0.05$
Question 13	28 (34)	55 (66)	58 (26)	169 (74)	2.0 $p>0.05$
Question 15	9 (11)	74 (89)	54 (24)	172 (76)	6.4 $p<0.05$

[a] Includes 'Not sure' and 'Not applicable' responses.

organisational issues and those assessing the basis used for formulating the guidelines.

The results suggest that many of the guidelines in the study were developed through *ad-hoc* methodologies without a rigorous approach. In particular, the methods used for searching and assessing the evidence were judged generally inadequate, as were the techniques for formulating the recommendations. Likewise, the linkage between final recommendations and underlying evidence was often opaque. Secondly, guidelines produced by national groups tended to be more rigorously developed than local ones. Thirdly, recently developed guidelines performed better, suggesting that recent guidance on guideline development is being assimilated. Until 1993 there had been little guidance on how guidelines should be developed. Since then, the principles for developing 'good' guidelines have been widely disseminated in the UK[16] and potential guideline developers are encouraged to follow them.[51] To ensure that valid guidelines are promulgated it is likely to be more cost-effective to concentrate on creating a few evidence-based national guidelines that can act as templates, rather than to advocate widespread guideline development. Local efforts should be re-targeted at guideline adaptation, dissemination and implementation.[8]

An important outcome from this research programme has been that the instrument is currently used to appraise national guidelines as part of the NHS guideline appraisal programme. This provides a basis to decide on which guidelines to use in practice. It also enables the regular reviewing of the instrument by adding the results from the appraised guidelines to the research base.

References

1 Robertson JI (1994) Guidelines for the treatment of hypertension: a critical review. *Cardiovascular Drugs and Therapy*, **8**(4): 665–72.

2 Joint National Committee on Detection and Treatment of High Blood Pressure (1993) The Fifth Report of the Joint National Committee on Detection and Treatment of High Blood Pressure (JNC V). *Archives of Internal Medicine*, **153**: 154–83.

3 Sever P, Beevers G, Bulpitt C, Lever A, Ramsay L, Reid J and Swales J (1993) Management guidelines in essential hypertension: report of the second working party of the British Hypertension Society. *BMJ*, **306**: 983–7.

4 Myers MG, Carruthers SG, Leenen FH and Haynes RB (1989) Recommendations from the Canadian Hypertension Society Consensus Conference on the Pharmacologic Treatment of Hypertension. *Canadian Medical Association Journal*, **140**: 1141–6.

5 Jackson R, Barham P, Bills J, Birch T, McLennan L, MacMahon S and Maling T (1993) Management of raised blood pressure in New Zealand: a discussion document. *BMJ*, **307**: 107–10.

6 Subcommittee of WHO/ISH Mild Hypertension Liaison Committee (1993) Summary of 1993 World Health Organisation – International Society of Hypertension Guidelines for the Management of Mild Hypertension. *BMJ*, **307**: 1541–6.

7 Fahey TP and Peters TJ (1996) What constitutes controlled hypertension? Patient based comparison of hypertension guidelines (see comments). *BMJ*, **313**: 93–6.

8 Thomson R, McElroy H and Sudlow M (1998) Guidelines on anticoagulant treatment in atrial fibrillation in Great Britain: variation in content and implications for treatment. *BMJ*, **316**: 509–13.

9 Jackson RT and Sackett DL (1996) Guidelines for managing raised blood pressure. *BMJ*, **313**: 64–5.

10 Swales JD (1994) Guidelines for management of hypertension. Sticking to guidelines can be expensive. *BMJ*, **308**: 855.

11 Sheldon TA and Smith GD (1993) Consensus conferences as drug promotion (letter). *Lancet*, **341**: 499.

12 McKee M and Clarke A (1995) Guidelines, enthusiasms, uncertainty, and the limits to purchasing (review). *BMJ*, **310**: 101–4.

13 Hopkins A (1995) Some reservations about clinical guidelines. *Archives of Disease in Childhood*, **72**: 70–5.

14 Paccaud F (1997) Variation in guidelines (a viewpoint on the paper by Fahey and Peters). *Journal of Health Services Research and Policy*, **2**: 53–5.

15 National Health Service Centre for Reviews and Dissemination (1994) *Effective Health Care. Implementing Clinical Practice Guidelines: Can Guidelines be Used to Improve Clinical Practice?* NHS CRD, University of York.

16 Grimshaw J, Eccles M and Russell I (1995) Developing clinically valid practice guidelines. *Journal of Evaluation in Clinical Practice*, **1**: 37–48.

17 Grimshaw JM and Russell IT (1994) Achieving health gain through clinical guidelines: II. Ensuring guidelines change medical practice. *Quality in Health Care*, **3**: 45–52.

18 Kendrick T (1997) Prescribing antidepressants in general practice. *BMJ*, **313**: 829–30.

19 Littlejohns P, Collier J and Hilton S (1992) Guidance on guidelines. *BMJ*, **305**: 1098.

20 Lohr KN and Field MJ (1992) A provisional instrument for assessing clinical practice guidelines. In: MJ Field and KN Lohr (eds) *Guidelines for Clinical Practice. From Development to Use*. Institute of Medicine/National Academy Press, Washington DC.

21 Field MJ and Lohr KN (eds) (1990) *Clinical Practice Guidelines: Directions for a New Program. Committee to Advise the Public Health Service on Clinical Practice Guidelines, Institute of Medicine*. National Academy Press, Washington DC.

22 Hayward RS, Wilson MC, Tunis SR, Bass EB and Guyatt G (1995) Users' guides to the medical literature: VIII. How to use clinical practice guidelines: A. Are the recommendations valid? The Evidence-Based Medicine Working Group. *JAMA*, **274**: 570–4.

23 Baker R and Fraser RC (1995) Development of review criteria: linking guidelines and assessment of quality. *BMJ*, **311**: 370–3.

24 Cluzeau F, Littlejohns P, Grimshaw J and Hopkins A (1995) Appraising clinical guidelines and the development of criteria: a pilot study. *Journal of Interprofessional Care*, **9**: 227–35.

25 Hayward RS, Wilson MC, Tunis SR, Bass EB, Rubin HR and Haynes RB (1993) More informative abstracts of articles describing clinical practice guidelines. *Annals of Internal Medicine*, **118**: 731–7.

26 Cluzeau F, Littlejohns P and Grimshaw J (1994) Appraising clinical guidelines – towards a 'which' guide for purchasers. *Quality in Health Care*, **3**: 121–2.

27   Lichtenstein S, Slovic P, Fischhoff B, Layman M and Comb B (1978) Judged frequency of lethal events. *Journal of Experimental Psychology: Human Learning and Memory*, **4**: 551–78.

28   Haynes RB (1993) Some problems in applying evidence in clinical practice (discussion, 224–5). *Annals of the New York Academy of Sciences*, **703**: 210–24.

29   Feder G (1994) Clinical guidelines in 1994. *BMJ*, **309**: 1457–8.

30   Clinical Resource and Audit Group (1993) *Clinical Guidelines*. The Scottish Office, Edinburgh.

31   Oxman AD, Guyatt GH, Singer J, Goldsmith CH, Hutchison BG, Milner RA and Streiner DL (1991) Agreement among reviewers of review articles. *Journal of Clinical Epidemiology*, **44**: 91–8.

32   Leape L, Park RE, Kahan JP and Brook RH (1992) Group judgements of appropriateness: The effect of panel composition. *Quality Assurance in Health Care*, **4**: 151–9.

33   Scott EA and Black N (1991) When does consensus exist in expert panels? *Journal of Public Health Medicine*, **13**: 1317–20.

34   Fink A, Kosecoff J, Chassin M and Brook RH (1984) Consensus methods: characteristics and guidelines for use. *American Journal of Public Health*, **74**: 979–83.

35   Siverg B (1993) *Professional Judgement. A Theoretical Model and Multi-experiments in Nursing Professional Judgement*. Lund University Press, Sweden.

36   Cluzeau F, Littlejohns P, Grimshaw J and Feder G (1997) *Appraisal Instrument for Clinical Guidelines Version 1*. St. George's Hospital Medical School, London.

37   Eddy DM (1990) Clinical decision making: from theory to practice. Guidelines for policy statements: the explicit approach. *JAMA*, **263**: 2239–43.

38   Keeley D and Rees J (1997) New guidelines on asthma management. *BMJ*, **314**: 315.

39   Eccles M, Clapp Z, Grimshaw J, Adams PC, Higgins B, Purves I and Russell I (1996) Developing valid guidelines: methodological and procedural issues from the North of England Evidence Based Guideline Development project. *Quality in Health Care*, **5**: 44–50.

40   Eccles M, Clapp Z, Grimshaw J, Adams C, Higgins B, Purves I and Russell I (1996) North of England Evidence Based Guideline Development Project: methods of guideline development. *BMJ*, **312**: 760–2.

41   Jones J and Hunter D (1995) Consensus methods for medical and health services research. *BMJ*, **311**: 376–80.

42   Woolf SH (1994) An organized framework for practice guideline

development: Using the analytic logic as a guide for reviewing evidence, developing recommendations, and explaining the rationale. In: KM McCormick, S Moore and RA Siegel, (eds) *Clinical Practice Guideline Development: Methodology Perspectives*. Agency for Health Care Policy and Research/US Department of Health and Human Services, Rockville, MD.

43 Baker R and Feder G (1997) Clinical guidelines: Where next? *International Journal for Quality in Health Care*, **9**: 399–404.

44 Wilson MC, Hayward RS, Tunis SR, Bass EB and Guyatt G (1995) User's guides to the medical literature: VIII. How to use clinical practice guidelines: B. What are the recommendations and will they help you in caring for your patients? The Evidence Based Medicine Working Group. *JAMA*, **274**: 1630–2.

45 Rigge M (1996) The changing role of the consultant physician: What sort of doctor? *Journal of the Royal College of Physicians of London*, **30**: 505–8.

46 Feder G, Griffiths C, Highton C, Eldridge S, Spence M and Southgate L (1995) Do clinical guidelines introduced with practice based education improve care of asthmatic and diabetic patients? A randomised controlled trial in general practices in east London. *BMJ*, **311**: 1473–8.

47 Mitman BS, Tonesk X and Jacobson PD (1992) Implementing clinical guidelines: social influence strategies and practitioner behaviour change. *Quality Review Bulletin*, **18**: 413–22.

48 Cluzeau F, Littlejohns P, Grimshaw J and Feder G (1997) National survey of UK guidelines for the management of coronary heart disease, lung and breast cancer, asthma and depression. *Journal of Clinical Effectiveness*, **2**: 120–3.

49 Oxman AD and Guyatt GH (1991) Validation of an index of the quality of review articles. *Journal of Clinical Epidemiology*, **44**: 1271–8.

50 Streiner DL and Norman GR (1995) *Health Measurement Scales. A Practical Guide to Their Development and Use* (2e). Oxford University Press, New York.

51 National Health Service Executive (1996) *Clinical Guidelines: Using Clinical Guidelines to Improve Patient Care Within the NHS*. NHS Executive, Leeds.

Appendix: Appraisal instrument

Dimension 1 Rigour of development process

1 Is the agency responsible for the development of the guidelines clearly identified?

2 Was external funding or other support received for developing the guidelines?

3 If external funding or support was received, is there evidence that the potential biases of the funding body(ies) were taken into account?

4 Is there a description of the individuals (e.g. professionals, interest groups – including patients) who were involved in the guidelines development group?

5 If so, did the group contain representatives of all key disciplines?

6 Is there a description of the sources of information used to select the evidence on which the recommendations are based?

7 If so, are the sources of information adequate?

8 Is there a description of the method(s) used to interpret and assess the strength of evidence?

9 If so, is (are) the method(s) for rating the evidence adequate?

10 Is there a description of the methods used to formulate the recommendations?

11 If so, are the methods satisfactory?

12 Is there an indication of how the views of interested parties not on the panel were taken into account?

13 Is there an explicit link between the major recommendations and the level of supporting evidence?

14 Were the guidelines independently reviewed prior to the publication/release?

15 If so, is explicit information given about the methods and how comments were addressed?

16 Were the guidelines piloted?

17 If so, is explicit information given about the methods used and the results adopted?

18 Is there a mention of a date for reviewing or updating the guidelines?

19 Is the body responsible for the reviewing and updating clearly identified?

20 Overall, have the potential biases of guideline development been adequately dealt with?

Dimension 2 Context and content

21 Are the reasons for developing the guidelines clearly stated?

22 Are the objectives of the guidelines clearly defined?

23 Is there a satisfactory description of the patients to which the guidelines are meant to apply?

24 Is there a description of the circumstances (clinical or non-clinical) in which exceptions might be made in using the guidelines?

25 Is there an explicit statement of how the patient's preferences should be taken into account *in applying the guidelines*?

26 Do the guidelines describe the condition to be detected, treated, or prevented in unambiguous terms?

27 Are the different possible options for the management of the condition clearly stated in the guidelines?

28 Are the recommendations clearly presented?

29 Is there an adequate description of the health benefits that are likely to be gained from the recommended management?

30 Is there an adequate description of the potential harms or risks that may occur as a result of the recommended management?

31 Is there an estimate of the costs or expenditures likely to incur from the recommended management?

32 Are the recommendations supported by the estimated benefits, harms and costs of the intervention?

Dimension 3 Application of guidelines

33 Does the guideline document suggest possible methods for dissemination and implementation?

34 (*National guidelines only*) Does the guideline document identify key elements which need to be considered by local guideline groups?

35 Does the guideline document specify criteria for monitoring compliance?

36 Does the guideline document identify clear standards or targets?

37 Does the guideline document define measurable outcomes that can be monitored?

7
Setting national guidelines in a local context

Allen Hutchinson and Gene Feder

A great deal of time has been spent by health service professionals in developing local clinical guidelines. The advent of national evidence-based clinical guidelines has provided an opportunity to save effort on assembling evidence and constructing recommendations, but there remains an argument for local adaptation of national guidelines. In this chapter, the authors review the value of local adaptations, examine the purpose of local adaptation and consider the best approaches. Examples of national and local guideline recommendations are used as a basis for the discussion.

Introduction

Nationally produced clinical guidelines can be used as the basis for local guidelines and clinical standards that are sensitive to local circumstances. In this chapter, we examine the potential benefits of converting national guidelines to local guidelines, what the differences between national and local guidelines might be, and how conversion might best be managed.

In the coming years, national clinical practice guidelines will become methodologically sounder and more valid. They will be based on systematic assessments of the best available evidence, will have multidisciplinary input and will be led by professional associations such as Nederlands Huisarten Genootschap (NHG) in the Netherlands or the medical and nursing Royal Colleges in the UK. Alternatively, they may be sponsored by government agencies such as the Agency for Health Care Policy and Research (AHCPR) in the US and by regional health departments – for instance, the Australian New South Wales Health Department which was responsible for a 1996 evidence-based consensus guideline on diabetes.[1]

The case is stronger than ever for producing national clinical guidelines, rather than overwhelming health professionals with a raft of locally produced guidelines of varying provenance. There is a substantial efficiency argument for creating evidence-based guidelines on a national level, with the emphasis on drawing together scarce methodological resources and the ability to access evidence from relatively inaccessible sources. This avoids reduplication of effort in scores of different settings such as hospitals, quality groups and office or general practice, with no one group quite knowing what the others are doing.

Efficiency in guideline production is an important issue. After all, it takes considerable effort and substantial resources in terms of finance and people with special skills to develop a national guideline. Sums of up to $500 000 to $1 million have been quoted for some of the more substantial guidelines developed in the US and it is becoming clear that the true cost of national guideline production in the UK can be of the order of £200 000 ($300 000). For instance, even though the national guideline for acute back pain[2] (*see also* Chapter 2) was based mainly on existing evidence reviews, and additional reviews were limited to specific areas, such as the effectiveness of bedrest, it still cost approximately £60 000 ($90 000) in new resources. Even then, the substantial costs of contributors' time was given 'free of charge'.

However, in the broader sense of efficiency, it could be argued that it is the effective use of guidelines at the local level, with appropriate improvements in quality of care, where the real efficiencies of guidelines are to be found. In this chapter, therefore, we explore the value of converting national guidelines into local versions which reflect the context of care and local services, and consider what approaches might be used in bringing together appropriate national and local components.

The argument for creating local versions of national guidelines has three planks:

1 the structure, orientation and priorities of the guideline

2 the value of local ownership of the work

3 the setting of the guidelines into a local context.

Structure, orientation and priorities in guideline setting

Clinical guidelines should aim to be valid and reliable[3] through a robust and transparent process which is quality assured (e.g. *see* Chapter 6). But in addition to the quality of the content, increased attention is now being given to structure of the guidelines so that they are usable by the target groups of professionals or patients. So, in addition to an evidence base and its attendant recommendations (which are often rather weighty tomes), national guidelines may now have a summary, perhaps just one page, which is designed to be easily accessible to the practising clinician in a busy workplace.

But there are limitations to the 'one size fits all' national format and approach. It is almost by definition a rather abstract document, since it is usually oriented to a national, population perspective rather than to a locality or health district, and the recommendations usually lack specificity as to roles and responsibilities.

Take, for instance, the advice given in the well-respected guidelines entitled *Making the Best Use of a Department of Clinical Radiology*.[4] The information is designed for doctors in both primary and hospital care, of varying degrees of training and experience and working in very different settings. So, the language is formal and concise and the recommendations are generic, based on general population data rather than related to the clinician's local population. Table 7.1 is an example adapted from the section on the cervical spine (p. 31).[4]

Priority choices may also be required because of resource constraints, spending priorities in particular localities or specific local concerns and interests. Although the implementation of recommendations from a clinical guideline may not necessarily require additional funding (the Royal College of Radiologists guidelines are intended to conserve resources), increased costs may well flow from guideline implementation. Local judgement on what is affordable may be both pragmatic and an essential part of the implementation process. Guidelines which recommend, for example, diagnostic tests which are not funded locally will lose credibility with clinicians.

Priority choices may also be made on the basis of addressing topics that have particular local significance. Since time and human resources must be given to implementation, decisions that focus on specific topics within a guideline and which are seen as especially relevant by clinicians and managers may substantially increase interest in implementing

Table 7.1: Cervical spine X-ray guidelines – an example (adapted from Royal College of Radiologists[4])

Clinical problem	Investigation	Guideline	Comment
Neck pain: ?degenerative disease	XR	Six Week Suggestion	Usually due to disk/ ligamentous changes undetectable on plain XR. MRI increasingly being used, especially when brachalgia is present. Degenerative changes begin in early middle-age and are often unrelated to symptoms.
	MRI	Specialised investigation	Consider MRI and specialist referral when pain affecting lifestyle or when there are neurological signs. Myelography (with CT) may occasionally be required to provide further delineation or when MRI not available or impossible.

recommendations. For instance, in one local health authority in England, attention was focused on only three of six areas of recommendation in the national acute low back pain guideline.[2] These were:

1 reduction in lumbo-sacral spine X-ray – limited effectiveness in most cases

2 early mobility – to reduce limitation of mobility

3 early access to physical therapy – reduction of proportion of chronic cases.

Ownership

Achieving local ownership of a guideline is sometimes regarded as the key to getting the evidence contained in guidelines introduced into practice. Some clinical staff are said to be more likely to take notice of the evidence and the recommendations contained in the guideline if they or close colleagues have been involved in producing it. Results from the North of England Study on Standards and Performance in General Practice, undertaken in the 1980s, tend to support this view.[5]

Much effort seems to have been expended on local guideline development as a result of this thesis, yet the evidence of the importance of local ownership seems to be equivocal. For instance, Canadian researchers Puttnam and Curry found that local ownership of guidelines had a positive influence on the uptake of the recommendations in respect of improvements of patient care in one study[6] but not in another.[7] In British clinical practice, the large North of England Study on Standards and Performance in General Practice[5] was able to demonstrate the value of local ownership both in the expressed opinions of the doctors concerned and through changes in the process of care provided for children. Doctors in teaching practices who had put considerable effort into developing local clinical standards were much more likely to change their practice for topics on which they had been involved than for topics on which their colleagues across the region had done the development work. However, more recently there is evidence that the postal dissemination of guidelines in the south-west of London (i.e. without ownership by the target clinicians) was successful in changing clinician behaviour.[8]

It is probable that there is a complex play of interactions in relation to the value of local contributions to guidelines leading to greater ownership, and subsequently to more effective adoption of the guideline recommendations. For some health professionals the variations in responses to guidelines, together with an individual professional's view that a personal contribution is required before adoption, will be associated with the individual way in which clinicians learn. What may be an effective method of accessing and adopting new information into practice for one professional may not be effective for another.[9] There is some evidence to suggest that learning methods differ greatly and that, therefore, there can be no one standardised method which can apply to the great majority of learners.

The concept of 'ownership' may be inappropriate for an understanding of why clinicians adopt some guidelines and not others. Thus, for some clinicians the requirement may not be for involvement in the development of guidelines *de novo*, but for involvement at some time before dissemination or a decision to implement. Others might wish to be involved with development before accepting recommendations whereas others are content to use materials which are seen to have a good pedigree. A local approach which takes account of these varying requirements may have a greater chance of attracting local support.

Context

A real issue for the effective implementation of guidelines is the physical and organisational context in which clinicians work, since the settings vary dramatically from one to another. This applies not just between obviously different contexts such as those of primary and secondary care. The variation in physical and organisational terms, and the resource levels available to undertake new initiatives, can be almost as great between hospitals or between general practice or specialist office practice.

Premises can vary in quality from the venerable to the ultramodern. The ethnic and sociodemographic mix of the local population may be dramatically different between one setting and another, particularly in general practice. Also, the resources available to treat patients differ between localities or regions and countries. For instance, in 1996 the health service in Scotland had at least 12% more resources per head of the population than did the NHS in England.

Fitting recommendations to local resources and concerns, while retaining the link to underlying evidence, is likely to increase the impact of guidelines on practice (although we do not yet have empirical evidence for this supposition) (*see* Box 7.1).

Box 7.1: A local guideline example

In east London, developers of guidelines on the primary care management of dyspepsia were faced with the absence of any *Helicobacter pylori* testing in one of the localities. The health authority was persuaded to commission an *H. pylori* serology service which made testing a feasible strategy. *Helicobacter pylori* breath-testing was not available in any of the localities and did not figure in the guidelines, particularly as evidence for its usefulness over and above serology was debatable.

A similar contextualising approach might be taken with the orientation of a guideline. As Eccles and his colleagues describe in Chapter 3, the questions which a guideline will address are driven by national public health policy issues and may address a considerable agenda. For local requirements, however, only a subset of the guideline might be necessary, perhaps because a priority has been given to a particular aspect of clinical practice. In the UK, for example, much use has been made in general practice of the section of the Royal College of

Radiologists guidelines relating to the use of radiology in the management of acute back pain.

All of these differences provide challenges for the implementation of national clinical guidelines, since the barriers which some contexts put in the way of good practice may seem insuperable (maintaining the quality of care under the pressures of inner city practice, for instance). Yet equity of access to good care, informed by the best available evidence, is a goal of all developed healthcare systems and clinical practice guidelines exist to support good quality care. So how may local versions of national guidelines assist this purpose and what criteria should guide the content of the local version?

Making the decision

It is neither mandatory nor always necessary to spend time converting national guidelines. For some clinical settings or conditions, the context of practice may be relatively similar and the type of care relatively standardised, so that application of national recommendations is straightforward in professional terms (although whether the appropriate resources are available may be another matter entirely!).

Although one of the criticisms of guidelines is that they may 'standardise' health and medical care (an argument examined in Chapter 1), there is already a great deal of appropriate standardisation. For instance, although resource levels undoubtedly differ between hospitals, some guidelines for specialist services may well be applied in circumstances where the difference in context and facilities is relatively small, such as in aspects of cardiac surgery, the management of end-stage renal failure and in the pathology services (a specialty where benchmarking was first introduced in the UK).

Thus, the first criterion for choosing to create a local version of a national guideline is to determine whether the variation in settings is great enough to warrant local interpretation. This is particularly likely to be the case when care for patients is being considered which requires a multidisciplinary approach or where the care process crosses interfaces between, for instance, primary and secondary care or between health and social care.

The second criterion for choosing to develop a local version is the common need to prioritise changes in practice, either because there is a lack of resources to do everything at once or, just as likely, there is a local judgement that of the recommendations in a national guideline there are certain themes which are of particular local importance. Clearly, priority setting from among a set of recommendations in the national guideline requires a prior knowledge of where the local priority areas will be, probably based on a combination of clinical audit and knowledge of the structure and function of local health services.

A third factor in making the decision on whether to develop a local guideline version is the level of pressure for local involvement. Because, as we have already argued, the extent to which individual clinicians want to be involved in development is variable, a local discussion to determine strength of feeling is often a valuable first step. It may be that some health professionals in a locality prefer to use the national version while others want a local version. Congruity between the two versions is obviously essential to ensure common clinical practice across the locality, as well as ensuring that the guideline reflects the national evidence-based recommendations.

Who should decide whether a local version should be created? Context plays a part here too. In the British NHS it may be a partnership between clinical groups from different specialities. For example, the group might consist of nurses, cardiologists and accident and emergency specialists in the case of a guideline on the management of unstable angina in hospital. Whatever the setting, in whichever country, it is also probable that there will be input from health service management (since there is almost inevitably a resources issue to be addressed), even if only to find the resources to support the group's work. Management input may include contributions from the organisations that provide the financial resources for care, such as local health authorities or insurance companies. This is likely to be the case when the recommendations for a guideline cross between primary and secondary care, because of the increased management task of bringing the various parties together.

Increasingly, local patient groups and special interest groups will become a force in this process. Building on the experience of national guidelines for patients in the US, the national acute back pain project developed evidence-based information for patients,[10] and local ethnic minority newspapers printed versions of the clinical guideline. As locality commissioning becomes a reality in the NHS, patient groups will seek greater input into the guideline process. Already, some areas have developed patient versions of locally developed guidelines with the input of local patient groups. For example, in east London, patient versions of raised blood pressure and back pain guidelines reflect the multi-ethnic composition of the population.

Finally, someone will have to take local organisational responsibility, preferably an individual with experience in the collection and interpretation of evidence. In the UK this is often someone from a local public health department, university, or from a local quality or clinical audit group.

Rule 1: do not ignore the evidence-based recommendations

The greatest risk in creating local versions of guidelines is a tendency to rewrite the guideline in such a way as to reinterpret the evidence on which the recommendations are based (or to ignore it altogether!). The result may be a set of recommendations that are based on current local practice or local views of how practice ought to be, rather than on appropriate evidence.

Indeed, the tendency to base guidelines on incomplete or idiosyncratic versions of the evidence has, until recently, been a tendency of national guidelines so it is wrong to judge too harshly the work of local groups. But now that much effort is going into the evidence base of guidelines and that evidence and recommendations are being graded according to international standards, it would be dangerous for local groups to reinterpret recommendations where the evidence is strong without rigorously reappraising the original research papers.

However, there is still scope for local interpretation where evidence is weak or unobtainable. In the UK national guidance for breast cancer care, for example, a very strong evidence base was assembled by the Mario Negro Institute in Milan and the Centre for Reviews and Dissemination at the University of York.[11] For many of the clinical interventions the evidence was strong (graded 1 or 2 in a range of 1 to 4) and the associated recommendations were graded A or B (in a range of A to C). An example of a grade A recommendation is shown in Box 7.2.

Box 7.2: Radiotherapy effects on the recurrence of breast cancer

There is very strong evidence from a systematic review of randomised controlled trials that radiotherapy produces a significant overall reduction of 24% in local recurrence rates. This is particularly important for women who have breast-conserving surgery, which is associated with a considerably higher local recurrence rate than mastectomy (A).[11]

But in other areas of care, such as referral to hospital or care for recurrent disease, there was much weaker evidence (graded 3 or 4) and the recommendations were accordingly weaker in strength (graded C). Guidance of this nature may still be of value, but local interpretation may well be appropriate. An example of a grade C recommendation is shown in Box 7.3.

Box 7.3: Palliative care in breast cancer: continuity of care

There is no evidence showing an association between any specific organisational model and better continuity of care, but good communication between the palliative care team and the patient's GP may improve quality of care (C).[11]

Inevitably, given the gaps in the research base about whether new clinical interventions (or many long-established interventions) actually work in practice, there will always be recommendations which are relatively weak and which will be open to, and benefit from, local interpretation.

Local groups, local users, local versions

Local versions do not just create themselves. Someone has to take a hard-headed decision that such a project at least shows promise and that there is a local need and willingness to participate. The professional roles of the decision makers matter less than their ability to make a judgement of the benefits and costs of undertaking the project and their ability to cause the project to happen.

It is unlikely that a substantial project is worthwhile at an organisational level smaller than a hospital or a locality covering populations of under 200 000 to 300 000 people, for the costs in staff time are bound to be considerable. Furthermore, smaller projects which improve quality of care for one group of patients may create inequalities for those patients whose clinical teams are not part of the project. On the other hand, variation in access and quality remains a feature of all developed heath services so local projects may be valuable as demonstration projects. Local projects might also have a slightly different focus, such as adding clinical standards for individual teams to the national guideline. A key part of the decision-making process is to take account of these matters.

Local ownership (and the chances of success with local implementation) are best gained by a project which takes account of the key players, is multidisciplinary and is realistic about implementation in the light of available resources if change in practice requires new investment. Local versions of national guidelines therefore require input from clinicians from the relevant fields of medicine, nursing and professions allied to medicine, public health input to give the population perspective, and health service management to ensure policy and resource linkages.

Sometimes it may be necessary to seek assistance from staff who have experience in critical appraisal of evidence if the local version is derived a significant time after the national guideline is published. Updating of the evidence base may occasionally be required.

At a time when there are few national guidelines in the UK, local versions abound and it is not always easy to find a useful version to adopt. This situation has changed in a number of countries in the past decade with the establishment of national centres for improving quality such as CBO and NHG in the Netherlands, the Scottish Clinical Resource and Audit Group (CRAG) and Scottish Intercollegiate Guidelines Network (SIGN) in Scotland and the National Centre for Clinical Audit in England. These centres, together with increasing availability of materials on the Internet, will improve the access of local groups to versions which might save considerable effort.

Finally, a good project leader with competent group leadership skills is a great asset. Someone on the team with project management skills is similarly valuable.[12]

Local versions as clinical standards

Whether local versions of national guidelines are preferred, or the national version is to be used, there may be a role for a local group in developing a local standard to accompany the guideline. This may well be a rather different task from creating a local version, perhaps much better suited to a local quality group such as a clinical audit team. But it could also be developed by a local clinical team in a ward or a general practice. Certainly, the activity is much closer to implementation of the guideline than local refinement.

The purpose of adding standards to the guideline is to enable local targets to be met and evaluated during implementation. A recent, much worked, example is the local target setting for aspirin prescription in the secondary prevention of myocardial infarction. Recent research in the north of England shows that it still appears difficult to raise the level of aspirin to include almost all eligible patients (say 95%).[13] Many local quality groups are setting achievable, monitored standards to try to reach an appropriate treatment level in the population. An evidence-based example based on the north of England angina guideline[14] is shown in Box 7.4.

Box 7.4: Regular symptomatic treatment for people with angina of effort

Evidence-based statement: patients who have a myocardial infarction and are given beta blockers have a subsequently lower mortality rate (evidence grade 1 of range 1 to 3).[14]

Recommendation: all patients who require symptomatic treatment should be treated with a beta blocker (recommendation graded B because evidence extrapolated from the results of clinical trials).[14]

Local standard (which might apply to both hospital practice and general practice): 90% of people who have had a myocardial infarct and who require symptomatic therapy should be taking regular beta blocker treatment.

Local standards have three purposes. First, to take a very discrete component of practice and make its implementation an obvious priority. Secondly, to provide an achievable target which can be set differently for different groups at different times, but always with the aim of extending the target towards a locally agreed goal as teams reach their targets. There will almost always be reasons why targets cannot be 100%: guidelines are not compulsory protocols but take account of clinical circumstances and patient preferences, but for a therapy such as aspirin in coronary heart disease, a final target of 95% of patients is probably not unreasonable. Third, standards enable clinical teams to monitor the quality of their care in a form which they can compare with other similar teams.

Overall, there is a strong case for developing clinical standards from guidelines and the probability is that whenever a national guideline is published, a local group should give consideration to developing standards, whether or not a local version emerges.

Conclusion

As national guidelines become more commonplace, as they are, for instance, in the Netherlands, Scotland and to some extent in the US, it is probable that some of the current local guideline development activity will cease. The thrust of the argument in this chapter is that some clearly directed and rigorous local adaptation of national guidelines may replace some of the development work, to the improvement of local health services and quality of care for patients.

References

1 Liddle J (1996) *The Evidence for the NSW Health Department Guidelines for the Clinical Management of Diabetes Mellitus in Adults*. New South Wales Health Department, Sydney.
2 Waddell G, Feder G, McIntosh A, Lewis M and Hutchinson A (1996) *Low Back Pain Evidence Review*. Royal College of General Practitioners, London.
3 Grimshaw J and Russell IT (1993) Achieving health gain through clinical guidelines: I. Developing scientifically valid guidelines. *Quality in Health Care*, **2**: 243–8.
4 Royal College of Radiologists (1995) *Making the best use of a Department of Clinical Radiology*. RCR, London.
5 North of England Study of Standards and Performance in General Practice (1992). Medical audit in general practice. 1. Effects on doctors' clinical behaviour for common childhood conditions. *BMJ*, **304**: 1480–4.
6 Putnam R W and Curry L (1985) Impact of patient care appraisal on physician behaviour in the office setting. *Canadian Medical Association Journal*, **132**: 1025–9.
7 Putnam RW and Curry L (1989) Physicians' participation in establishing criteria for hypertension management in the office: Will patient outcomes be improved? *Canadian Medical Association Journal*, **140**: 806–9.
8 Oakeshott P, Kerry SM and Williams JE (1994) Randomised controlled trial of the effect of the Royal College of Radiologist's guidelines on general practitioners' referrals for radiographic examination. *British Journal of General Practitioners*, **44**: 197–200.
9 Vanhoorhees C, Wolf FM, Gruppen LD and Stross JK (1988) Learning Styles and Continuing Medical Education *Journal of Continuing Education in the Health Professions*, **8**: 257–65.
10 The Stationery Office (1996) *The Back Book*. HMSO, London.
11 National Health Service Executive (1996) *Improving Outcomes in Breast Cancer*. NHS Executive, Leeds.
12 Eccles M, Clapp Z, Grimshaw J, Adams PC, Higgins B, Purves I and Russell IT (1996). North of England Evidence Based Guidelines

Development Project: methods of guideline development. *BMJ*, **312**: 760–2.

13   Jones K, Wilson A, Russell I, Roberts A, O'Keeffe C, McAvoy B, Hutchinson A, Dowell A and Benech I (1996) Evidence based practice in primary care. *British Journal of the Community Health Nurse*, **1**: 276–80.

14   North of England Evidence-Based Guideline Development Project (1996) *Evidence-Based Clinical Practice Guideline: the primary care management of stable angina.* Report No. 75. Centre for Health Services Research, Newcastle-upon-Tyne.

8
Using guidelines to take evidence into practice

Ian Watt, Vicki Entwistle and Amanda Sowden

The goal of clinical practice guidelines is to improve the quality of healthcare provided to patients and, ultimately, health outcomes. For this to happen two things would seem to be necessary. First, guidelines need to be valid and based on the systematic identification and synthesis of research evidence of clinical and cost-effectiveness (*see* Chapter 6). Validity alone, however, is not sufficient to improve the quality of care and unless guidelines are actually followed in clinical practice, hoped for improvements will not occur. Thus, in any guideline initiative, attention needs to be paid not just to the development of guidelines, but also to their dissemination and implementation. This chapter discusses some of the issues that should be considered in introducing guidelines into clinical practice and ensuring adherence to their recommendations.

Introduction

The successful introduction of a clinical guideline is a complex process with three important stages: developing the guideline, educating clinicians about the guideline (through a process of dissemination) and ensuring they act upon the guideline (through implementation programmes).

Guideline development

This is discussed in detail in Chapters 2 and 3 and is only briefly mentioned here in the context of its potential impact on adherence to the guideline in practice.

Guidelines can be developed by groups including clinicians who will be using the guidelines in practice (end users), or by groups without end user representation.[1] It is often assumed that end-user involvement in guideline development, in part by increasing ownership, improves the implementation of guidelines (*see also* Chapter 7). However, a review of studies that addressed guideline implementation found only two of the four studies which considered the effects of ownership showed this to be the case.[2] The behavioural factors involved in the development of guidelines that influence adherence are very complex, and guidelines produced locally by professional end-users may at times be seen as less credible than those produced by locally respected clinicians or national experts.[3]

The development–implementation gap

The adoption of a particular guideline into practice will often necessitate a change of behaviour in the relevant healthcare professionals so that practices deemed by good research evidence to be less effective or cost-effective are replaced by those indicated by the guideline to be more effective. One traditional view of how such changes might be brought about is shown in Figure 8.1

Here, it is naïvely assumed that when a guideline is developed, it is somehow accessed by practitioners, appraised and then applied in daily practice. One established way in which guidelines have been communicated with clinicians has been through scientific journals, which has been shown on many occasions to be largely ineffective in influencing practice,[4] as has a process of simply mailing guidelines.[5] Yet, even when more active communication strategies have been employed, perhaps using a credible dissemination body (such as the relevant professional organisation) to package the guideline and target its distribution, the results in terms of appropriate changes in clinical practice have been largely disappointing.[4] There is, thus, a gap between guideline development and adoption into practice, the reasons for which can be broadly summarised below.

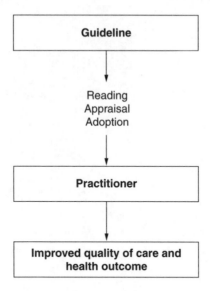

Figure 8.1   Adoption of a guideline: a traditional model.

The gap between guideline development and practice: potential barriers

The following are factors that may affect guideline development and practice:

- access to guideline
- environmental factors
- professional inertia
- perceived usefulness.

Although knowledge of a guideline may be important, it is rarely by itself sufficient to change practice, and a more realistic model than Figure 8.1 would refer to factors identified as important by the behavioural sciences and other knowledge bases. Lomas' co-ordinated implementation model,[6] for example, identifies a wide range of additional factors that can influence practice, such as the administrative, economic and community environment of the practitioner (*see* Figure 8.2). Also of importance are factors related to the clinician such as their individual beliefs and attitudes. For

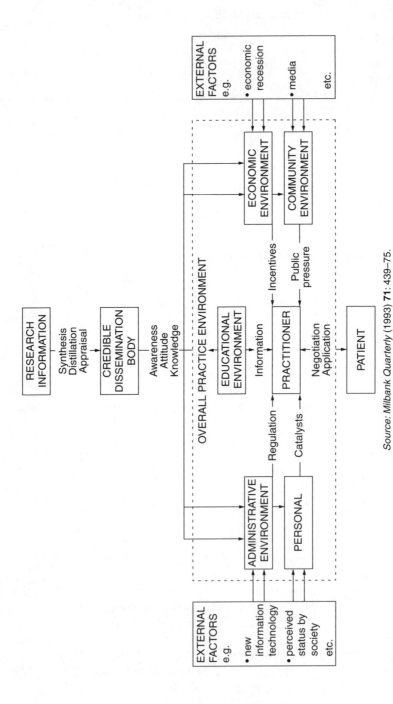

Figure 8.2 Adoption of a guideline: the co-ordinated implementation model.

Source: *Milbank Quarterly* (1993) **71**: 439–75.

example, a study carried out by Cohen *et al.*[7] to evaluate the effectiveness of a programme to increase adherence with preventive medicine guidelines found that in the intervention group (given age-specific checklists for preventive screening – attached to patient files and seminars), screening rates increased significantly relative to the control group. This was despite there being no significant differences in factual knowledge between intervention and control groups. However, there were significant differences in attitudinal scores, with the intervention physicians judging screening tests to be appropriate more frequently.

Dissemination

Lomas' implementation model does not remove the need for active dissemination, rather it places it in the context of the multitude of other factors to be considered in seeking to influence clinical practice. The literature on persuasive communication and advertising makes a distinction between communications that increase awareness and those that may actually bring about changes in behaviour.[8]

In attempting to introduce guidelines into practice both types of communication would seem to be necessary. As Lomas has stated, 'none of these programmes are likely to be successful if they are operating in a vacuum with no prior "predisposing" activities to make physicians aware of the information and prepare them to consider changes in practice'.[8] The NHS Centre for Reviews and Dissemination recognises that strategies to get research evidence adopted successfully into clinical practice should embrace a spectrum of activity which consists of dissemination activities at the one end, geared to raising awareness of research messages, to implementation activities at the other end that are more geared to getting the findings of research adopted into practice. While dissemination may be undertaken by national bodies and organisations, research evidence points to the importance of more local activities to promote implementation.[4,8]

The effectiveness of activities to disseminate clinical guidelines will be influenced by a number of factors,[9] including:

- source of communication
- media used
- audiences targeted.

Table 8.1 suggests a framework in which these concepts are interrelated between the processes of dissemination and implementation.

Table 8.1: Related concepts of dissemination and implementation of clinical guidelines

Dissemination	Implementation
←――――――→	
Communications to:	*Activities to:*
• raise awareness of research	• increase adoption of research findings
• facilitate readiness for change	• facilitate changes in practice
• help consideration of practice alternatives	• reinforce and support changes in practice

Implementation

A number of implementation strategies for clinical guidelines have been found to be at least partially effective (i.e. they have brought about some degree of change in the desired direction in the professional practice of the target group) and are outlined below. The difficulty, as will be discussed in more detail later in this chapter, is that no strategies have been shown to be successful in all circumstances,[10] and there is insufficient evidence to reach conclusions about the relative effectiveness of different implementation strategies in different contexts.

Potential implementation strategies

Audit and feedback

Formal audit of clinical practice is now part of most health professionals' working life. The process whereby actual practice is compared to agreed standards and the results fed back to practitioners can be an effective method of influencing their work and improving the quality of care. Clinical guidelines have been used to provide evidence-based audit standards, and a number of studies have shown that a process of audit and feedback can improve adherence to a guideline.[11,12] In one review of studies which had looked at the effects of audit/feedback, Mugford and colleagues[12] concluded that information feedback was most likely to influence clinical practice if it was part of a strategy to target decision makers who had already agreed to review their practice. They also stated that a more direct effect was discernible if the information was presented close to the time of decision making. Further insights into the influence of audit/feedback were given by Eisenberg[13] who stated that such approaches 'are most likely to be successful if the data are individualised, if doctors are compared with their peers, and if the information is delivered personally by a physician in a position of clinical leadership'.

Unfortunately, the potential value of clinical audit in changing professional practice as suggested by the above findings is often not utilised in the UK, where the feedback of audit results is often given in an anonymous manner and divorced from the time of decision making.

Educational outreach and academic detailing

Academic detailing (sometimes referred to as educational outreach) is based on activities begun by pharmaceutical sales representatives to market their products. It involves a face-to-face discussion with a credible individual supported by simple educational materials, in an informal setting during which the desired behaviour is outlined. A number of studies have shown academic detailing to be effective in influencing clinical practice from a non-commercial perspective.[10] In one study of academic detailers, two brief visits to physicians by clinical pharmacists trained in effective techniques of communication and persuasion as well as pharmacotherapy were found to significantly reduce inappropriate prescribing of a cerebral vasodilator, of cephalexin, and of propoxyphene by 14% in comparison with controls ($p = 0.0001$).[14] As well as pharmacists, academic detailers in studies have included physicians, standardised patients, study investigators, and nurse facilitators. Based on behavioural science theory and several field trials, Avorn and Soumerai identified[14] some of the most important techniques of 'detailing'. These include:[15]

1 conducting interviews to investigate health professionals' baseline knowledge and motivations for current practice

2 establishing credibility through a respected organisational identity, referencing authorative and unbiased sources of information, and presenting both sides of controversial issues

3 using concise graphic educational materials

4 highlighting and repeating the essential messages

5 providing positive reinforcement of improved practices (e.g. adherence to a clinical guideline) in follow-up visits.

Opinion leaders

Health workers, like many other professional groups, tend to operate more as closed communities than as collections of independent individuals.[16] Within such groups, individuals' decisions to follow a particular clinical policy or not may be based to a large extent on their perceptions of how their peers view the policy. Observation of what their colleagues are doing may influence both their awareness of new findings and their practice policies more than published articles.[17] In addition, research has shown that within a local community some people are more influential than others and exert a strong informal effect on the attitudes and behaviour of other members of the group. These people are often referred to as 'opinion leaders' or 'educational influentials', and their role in communities, as described in classical diffusion theory, is to evaluate new information in terms of group norms. In a study undertaken in the US, Hiss and colleagues investigated the personal characteristics which distinguished physician opinion leaders in community hospitals. The characteristics are summarised in the following three paragraphs, taken from Hiss and colleagues.[18]

They convey information in such a fashion as to provide a learning experience. They express themselves clearly and to the point – provide practical information first and then an explanation or rationale if time allows. They take the time to answer you completely and do not leave you with the feeling that they were too busy to answer your enquiry. They enjoy and are willing to share any knowledge they have.

They are individuals who like to teach. They are current and up to date and demonstrate a command of medical knowledge. They demonstrate a high level of clinical expertise.

They are 'caring' physicians who demonstrate a high level of humanistic concern. They never talk down to you, they treat you as an equal even though it's clear they are helping you.

Reminder systems

Some success in implementing guidelines has been found in the use of patient-specific reminders. In such approaches, contact with a patient initiates a specific reminder to the clinician to undertake an action suggested by the guideline. Reminders can either be designed to act during or outwith the consultation; they may also be manual or computerised. In their systematic review of methods to change physician performance, Davis and colleagues[10] found reminder systems to be an effective single method intervention in 22 out of 26 interventions reviewed. Four interventions in two studies failed to bring about any positive change in clinical practice. At their simplest, reminder systems may consist of nothing more than a structured sheet in the clinical notes which, if appropriately completed, would act as a prompt to specific actions. For example, such a sheet in the notes of all patients attending in a cardiology clinic might include a question about aspirin therapy. A study by Byme and colleagues[19] showed how the use of a structured formal risk assessment sheet in the notes of all general surgical admissions improved adherence to the hospital policy on the prophylaxis of venous thromboembolism. However, significant improvement was only achieved when the sheet was applied to the reverse of a standard prescription sheet and nurses given the task of informing house officers of their 'oversight' if it had not been completed. This example emphasises the importance of evaluating implementation strategies and 'fine-tuning' approaches in the light of local circumstances. More complex reminder strategies might involve the development of computer-based clinical decision support systems based on a specific guideline.[20]

Sharing clinical guidelines with patients

As well as disseminating clinical practice guidelines to relevant healthcare professionals, consideration may also be given to disseminating them, perhaps in a slightly modified form, to relevant patient groups and members of the public. Interest in providing patients with information about treatment options and their effects, and in involving patients more in decisions about their care, has increased in recent years. A succession of policy documents has reflected the assumption that greater patient involvement in treatment decisions is a 'good thing'.[21,22]

Patients have a vested interest in receiving appropriate, good quality healthcare, and there are plausible reasons to believe that sharing clinical practice guidelines with patients might help them influence the care they receive and prompt professional adherence to a guideline. Guidelines might inform patients about the available treatment options and about what forms of care are known to be effective.[23] Such information might be used by patients to help them input into decisions about the care they will receive, and to monitor the quality of care associated with a chosen intervention. (Similarly, beyond individual encounters, consumer representatives might use clinical guidelines when seeking to influence the prioritisation of healthcare services and clinical audit standards.)

The ability of an informed public to influence the clinical care they receive is suggested, for example, in a Swiss study[24] which describes the effect of a mass media campaign on hysterectomy rates. In the canton (county) where a public information programme about the rates of, and need for, hysterectomy took place, the annual rate of operations dropped by 26%, whereas in the reference canton, where no information was given to the public, hysterectomy rates increased by 1%. However, it is not clear from the study whether the media led this agenda or reflected it, and there is actually little empirical evidence on the effectiveness of using the media for encouraging guideline implementation.

Preference-flexible guidelines[25] (which are designed to incorporate the preferences of individual patients in clinical decisions) are more likely than preference-fixed guidelines (which provide generic treatment recommendations for patients with the same clinical indications) to facilitate patient involvement in decision making. The obvious advantage of preference-flexible guidelines is that they encourage the tailoring of decisions to individual preferences. This is more likely to be important when several treatment options with quite different outcome profiles might all be regarded as effective. Preference-fixed guidelines are likely to serve the more limited role of influencing patients' expectations of care and alerting them to any deviations in the care they receive from that which the guideline recommends. The format and presentation of clinical practice guidelines might need to be modified if they are to be understood by patients. A quick reference guide in technical shorthand might be ideal for busy health professionals, but unintelligible to the majority of patients. In addition, patients might want to know something of the rationale underlying the recommendations in the guideline; indeed, the guideline may not seem particularly credible without this.

The possible advantages of sharing clinical practice guidelines with patients include more informed patients, who might be able to use their knowledge to ensure they receive more effective (and possibly more appropriate) forms of care, which might in turn lead to greater health gain. In addition, some professional–patient relationships might benefit if communication about treatment is facilitated by the sharing of a guideline, and some patients might value opportunities presented by their possession of the guideline to become more involved in decisions about their care, and to assess the quality of the care they are given. However, it is not clear what proportion of patients, in what circumstances, will want or be able to change the behaviour of health professionals whose practice does not adhere to recommended guidelines. It is not clear whether a highly motivated, articulate and persuasive minority of patients will influence the care received by others as well as themselves.

The sharing of clinical guidelines with patients might generate outcomes which may be negatively valued if their use in practice does not lead to the advantages hoped for in theory. For example, it might lead to conflict between health professionals and patients, or to patient dissatisfaction with the process of care they receive. For the individual patients involved, this might impact adversely on their health status (although it may also lead to pressure for positive change). Sharing guidelines with patients may increase the likelihood of them being implemented, but it may also have a range of other effects, both positive and negative. Given our current state of understanding, it should therefore be seen as an intervention of uncertain consequences.

Theoretical issues

Very few of the studies that have assessed the effectiveness of strategies to disseminate and implement guidelines have explicitly identified the theoretical basis of the approaches used. This is not just of academic interest since an understanding of behaviour change theories may enhance the appropriateness of dissemination and implementation methods for specific situations and circumstances.

Many theories that have been developed to explain and predict behaviour change are relevant to the dissemination and implementation of clinical guidelines. They come from a wide range of disciplines including psychology, sociology, education and management. Important and relevant theoretical bodies of literature include:

- diffusion of innovations[26]
- social cognitive theory[27]
- social influences model[28]
- theory of learning and change[29]
- stages of change models (e.g. the trans-theoretical model)[30]
- social marketing[31]
- total quality management.[32]

It is beyond the scope of this chapter to discuss these and other theories in detail, and interested readers should refer to more specialised texts. As we note already, however, a knowledge of relevant theories encourages dissemination and enables implementation methods to be tailored to specific situations.

Ideally, the first stage of any strategy to implement a clinical guideline should be an information gathering exercise where an attempt is made to identify how current practice compares to that suggested by the guideline. If it diverges from the guideline's recommendation, prior information should also be gathered on people's 'readiness to change' and the potential barriers to successful guideline implementation.

For any particular behaviour change people may be at different stages, ranging from those who are not interested in considering change (often called pre-contemplators), through those uncertain about the prospect (contemplators) to those who are ready to change (preparation stage). Two further stages refer to those who have already embarked on change (the action and maintenance stages). This concept has been borrowed from the trans-theoretical model of behaviour change originally developed by Prochaska and DiClemente[30] to describe the processes involved in eliciting and maintaining change.

Along similar lines, an 'awareness-to-adherence' model of the steps to clinical guideline adoption has been reported. This model focuses on the cognitive and behavioural steps clinicians take when they adopt national clinical practice guidelines. Clinicians must first become aware of the guidelines, then intellectually agree with them, then decide to adopt them, then regularly adhere to them. This model was tested on survey data relating to national paediatric vaccine recommendations and was found to be generally accurate in describing the sequence of cognitive steps clinicians make when following clinical guidelines.[33]

In terms of barriers to change. Lomas' co-ordinated implementation model, discussed earlier in the chapter, has already indicated the wide range of influences that can have an impact on implementation.[6] In introducing a guideline the likely barriers to successful implementation should be assessed. It is important to consider the full range of individual, social, political and organisational influences that might exist in any given situation. It should not be automatically assumed, as is the case in many guideline implementation initiatives, that the main barrier to adoption of the guideline is a lack of knowledge in individual clinicians. For example, it may be a feeling of low self-efficacy that is the barrier to behaviour change. An individual would be expected to avoid a task that is felt to exceed their capabilities; therefore merely providing information would not aid in overcoming this particular barrier to change. Studies of guideline implementation that have included an assessment of specific barriers to change prior to deciding their implementation methods show high rates of positive changes in practice.[10]

Conclusion

Although there are gaps in our knowledge with respect to the effective dissemination and implementation of clinical guidelines, sufficient evidence exists to allow informed strategies to be developed. The first point to stress is that there is no blanket method that will lead to the universal adoption of guidelines in all situations and circumstances. Thus, any initiative to introduce a guideline in practice should start with an information-gathering exercise or 'needs assessment' among the target audience to identify current practice, relevant professionals' readiness to change and potential barriers to its successful adoption. Ideally, this exercise should begin early in the guideline's development and help inform its content in order to help make it as relevant as possible to the professional and patient groups concerned.

Once this first stage has been completed, an appropriate and co-ordinated strategy for dissemination and implementation can be planned. While dissemination can take place at a national and regional level, implementation activities are best undertaken as near as possible to the end user and integrated into the process of healthcare delivery. There is insufficient evidence to reach conclusions about the relative effectiveness of specific educational and implementation strategies in different contexts. Research suggests, however, that a dissemination/ implementation strategy is more likely to be successful if it is multi-faceted, rather than relying on a single approach. Guidelines should be disseminated to all relevant audiences and followed up by communications to reinforce the recommendations. The reinforcement might come from a number of different sources (e.g. professional bodies, purchasers, consumer groups). These educational and awareness-raising activities should be closely co-ordinated with the implementation methods used. The nature and number of implementation methods used will be determined, at least in part, by the resources available and the preliminary 'needs assessment'. The choice of implementation strategy should be guided by the characteristics of the guideline's message, recognition of barriers to change, and the stages of change of targeted clinicians.

Finally, the success or otherwise of dissemination/implementation activity should be monitored to allow whichever approach is used to be amended as necessary. It is important that we continue to add to our knowledge of how to successfully introduce guidelines into practice. Without this, the effort that goes into the development of valid clinical guidelines will be in danger of being wasted.

References

1   Grimshaw JM and Russell IT (1994) Achieving health gain through clinical guidelines: II. ensuring guidelines change medical practice. *Quality in Health Care*, **3**: 45–52.
2   National Health Service Centre for Reviews and Dissemination (1994) *Effective Health Care Implementing Clinical Practice Guidelines*. NHS CRD, University of York.
3   Sommers LS, Sholtz R, Shepherd RM *et al.* (1984) Physician involvement in quality assurance. *Medical Care*, **22**: 1115–38.
4   Kanouse D, Kallich D and Kahan JP (1995) Dissemination of effectiveness and outcomes research. *Health Policy*, **34**: 167–92.
5   Freemantle N, Harvey E, Grimshaw J, Wolf F, Oxman A, Grilli R and Bero L (1997) The effectiveness of printed educational materials in changing the behaviour of healthcare professionals. In: *The Cochrane Database of Systematic Reviews*. The Cochrane Collaboration, Oxford.
6   Lomas J (1993) *Teaching Old (and not so old) Dogs New Tricks: Effective Ways to Implement Research Findings*. Paper 93–4. Centre for Health Economics and Policy Analysis, McMaster University, Hamilton, Ontario.
7   Cohen DI, Littenberg B, Wetzel C and Neuhauser DB (1982) Improving physician compliance with preventive medicine guidelines. *Medical Care*, **20**: 1040–5.
8   Lomas J (1993) Retailing research: increasing the role of evidence in clinical services for child birth. *Millbank Quarterly*, **71**: 439–75.
9   McQuail D (1984) *Communication* (2e). Longman, London.
10 Davis DA, Thomson MA, Oxman A and Haynes B (1995) Changing physician performance, a systematic review of the effect of continuing medical education strategies. *JAMA*, **274**: 700–5.
11 Buntinx F, Winkens R, Grol R *et al.* (1993) Influencing diagnostic and preventive performance in ambulatory care by feedback and reminders: a review. *Family Practice*, **10**: 219–28.
12 Mugford M, Banfield P and O'Hanlon M (1991) Effects of feedback of information on clinical practice: a review. *BMJ*, **303**: 398–402.

13 Eisenberg J (1986) *Doctors Decisions and the Costs of Medical Care.* Administrative Press, Ann Arbor, MI.

14 Avorn J and Soumerai SB (1983) Improving drug therapy decisions through education outreach: a randomised controlled trial of academically based "detailing". *NEJM*, **308**: 1457–63.

15 Soumerai SB and Avorn J (1990) Principles of educational outreach ('Academic Detailing') to improve clinical decision making. *JAMA*, **263**: 549–56.

16 Greer AL (1988) The state of the art versus the state of the science: the diffusion of new medical technologies into practice. *International Journal of Technology Assessment in Health Care*, **4**: 5–26.

17 Horder J, Bosanquet N and Stocking B (1986) Ways of influencing the behaviour of general practitioners. *Journal of the Royal College of General Practitioners*, **36**: 517–21.

18 Hiss RG, MacDonald R and David WR (1978) Identification of physician educational influentials in small community hospitals. *Research in Medical Education*, **17**: 283–8.

19 Byme GJ, McCarthy MJ and Silverman SH (1996) Improving uptake of venous thromboembolism in general surgical patients using prospective audit. *BMJ*, **313**: 917.

20 Johnston ME, Langton KB, Haynes B and Mathieu A (1994) Effects of computer-based clinical decision support systems on clinical performance and patient outcome. *Annals of Internal Medicine*, **120**: 135–42.

21 National Health Service Executive Letter (1995) **68**: *Priorities and Planning Guidance for 1996/97.* NHS Executive, London.

22 National Health Service Executive (1996) *Patient Partnership: Building a Collaborative Strategy.* NHS Executive, Leeds.

23 Duff LA, Kelson M, Marriott S, McIntosh A, Brown S, Cape J, Marcus N and Traynor M (1996) Involving patients and users of services in quality improvement: what are the benefits? *Journal of Clinical Effectiveness*, **1**: 63–7.

24 Domenighetti G, Lurasch P, Casabianca A, Gatzwiller F, Spinelli A, Pedrinis E and Repetto F (1988) Effect of information campaign by the mass media on hysterectomy rates. *Lancet* **II**: 1470–3.

25 Nease RF and Owens DK (1994) A method for estimating the cost-effectiveness of incorporating patient preferences into practice guidelines. *Medical Decision Making*, **14**: 382–92.

26 Rogers E (1983) *Diffusion of innovations.* Free Press, New York.

27 Bandura A (1986) *Social Foundations of Thought and Action.* Prentice-Hall, Eaglewood Cliffs.

28 Mittman BS, Tonesk X and Jacobson PD (1992) Implementing

clinical practice guidelines: social influence strategies and practitioner behaviour change. *Quality Review Bulletin*, **18**: 413–22.

29 Fox RD, Mazmanian PE and Putnam RW (eds) (1989) *Changing and Learning in the Lives of Physicians.* Praeger, New York.

30 Prochaska JO and DiClemente CC (1982) Transtheoretical therapy: toward a more integrative model of change. *Psychotherapy: Theory, Research and Practice*, **19**: 276–88.

31 Kotler P (1984) Social marketing of health behaviour. In: LW Frederiksen, LJ Solomon and KA Brehony (eds) *Marketing Health Behaviour. Principles, Techniques and Applications.* Plenum Press, New York.

32 Berwick DM (1991) Controlling variation in healthcare: a consultation from Walter Showhart. *Medical Care*, **29**: 1212–25.

33 Palhman DE, Konrad TR, Freed GL, Freeman VH and Koch GG (1996) The awareness-to-adherence model of the steps to clinical guideline compliance. *Medical Care*, **34**: 873–89.

9
Taking research findings into practice: a collaborative model

Elaine Taylor-Whilde and Allen Hutchinson

Among a number of approaches to getting evidence into practice through implementing guideline recommendations, local frameworks to support changes in clinical practice have become increasingly popular. Often supported by investment from health authorities and health boards, clinical change programmes now combine guidelines set in a local health service context with systems for facilitating change. The guidelines initiative established by East Riding Health Authority in the north of England is used here as an example of a population-wide approach to improving the quality of care, incorporating evidence-based guidelines within a change agent-led facilitation programme. Innovative approaches include the use of consumer panels to work with professional groups in the design of local guidelines, audit projects and implementation of change.

Introduction

It is clear from the international research literature that one of the great barriers to improving the effectiveness of healthcare is the difficulty of taking research evidence into everyday clinical practice. The purpose of this chapter is to examine some of the methods and practical approaches that might be used to assist the assimilation of new research into practice. Based on some of the evidence-based approaches to implementation outlined in Chapter 8 and drawing on a range of models developed in settings other than direct patient care, for instance in manufacturing and service industries, it adds another dimension to the evidence-based commissioning initiatives referred to in Chapter 10.

Development and delivery of effective services is a key objective for everyone working in healthcare. In England a national policy on quality improvement started to emerge during the 1990s when the National Health Service Executive began to promote improvements in the effectiveness of clinical practice through a series of guidance documents,[1-3] directing the NHS to:

Improve the clinical and cost effectiveness of services throughout the NHS and thereby secure the greatest health gain from the resources available, through supporting R&D and formulating decisions on the appropriate evidence about clinical effectiveness.[3]

To provide an NHS-wide support for this process, a number of national centres for reviewing and disseminating information on effective practice were established (e.g. the Cochrane Centre in Oxford and the NHS Centre for Reviews and Dissemination in York), with the aim of enabling the whole range of clinicians and services to have easy access to up to date evidence relevant to their practice.

However, there is increasing research evidence to suggest that practitioner beliefs and attitudes to practice, rather than knowledge gaps, influence whether (and how quickly) evidence is incorporated into practice.[4] This provides special challenges for any group charged with the task of implementing evidence-based practice, especially when there may be differences in perception, beliefs and values between academics, managers and practitioners, who might have to work together to encourage the adoption of evidence-based practice. These differences in perception may actually create obstacles when implementing the recommendations contained within clinical practice guidelines (*see* Box 9.1).

Box 9.1: Examples of differences in perception when implementing guidelines

- the nature of the proposed change (e.g. the guideline users do not believe that the recommendations are feasible)

- organisational features of the care provider (poor motivation perhaps, or low skill levels)

- problems concerned with the interface between different sectors of the health service (e.g. lack of communication, or no supporting structures).

From theory to practice: an evidence-based local model

A number of studies from Western Europe and North America are indicating that 'evidence into practice' approaches which use multiple methods to enable behaviour change – the so-called multifaceted approach – offer the best chance of success (e.g. *see* Grimshaw and Russell[5] and Chapter 8). In the Netherlands, Grol[6] has used a step-by-step analysis of the barriers to change followed by the selection of appropriate interventions adapted to each obstacle to implement change, which was further adapted after evaluation. In the UK, Kitson developed a model for nursing practice based on the Canadian work of Lomas,[7] emphasising the importance of using change agents and a marketing approach to enable and reinforce behaviour change.

Popular among these developments in the UK have been initiatives to enable clinical teams and health authorities to take good quality clinical guidelines and tailor them for application locally. There are a number of models in existence, including the national King's Fund Promoting Action on Clinical Effectiveness (PACE) initiative[8] and the Oxford region GRiPP project (Getting Research into Practice and Purchasing[9]). Here we describe an example of a local implementation programme from the north of England, the East Riding Guidelines Initiative, as a means of examining a range of different approaches to getting evidence into practice, particularly focusing on methods based on the management sciences.

The East Riding Guidelines Initiative

Recognising the need to provide local support structures to help clinicians access evidence and adopt new practice, East Riding Health Authority and the local primary care quality group (the Hull and East Riding Multidisciplinary Audit Advisory Group) (MAAG) formed a partnership for an experimental two-year period in 1995. The aim of the partnership was to deliver evidence-based healthcare into practice in clinical priority areas, with a secondary objective of shifting resources away from ineffective care towards care of proven effectiveness. If successful, the sponsors hoped the project would:

- improve clinical outcomes
- maximise the use of resources
- improve patient, professional and commissioner (health authority) satisfaction.

The proposed methods of working were based on research evidence concerned with changing clinical behaviour, with the focus on creating local knowledge-based organisations capable of improving their own evidence-based healthcare approaches. Through its working practices the project would therefore test assumptions concerning the most effective methods of implementing clinical guidelines.

Two approaches were taken to developing an evidence base to support local implementation methods. Reviews of the literature on guideline implementation were accessed, particularly those of Oxman,[4] Grimshaw and Russell[5] and the Royal College of General Practitioners.[10] In addition, critical appraisal methods[11] were used to synthesise current research from management sciences concerning the management of change, from which were drawn six key success criteria for enhancing the chances of successful implementation of clinical guidelines:

1 a structured management process

2 well motivated professionals

3 top level commitment

4 investment of resources

5 key stakeholder involvement

6 involvement of all parts of the organisation.

Four particular pioneering approaches to changing NHS culture on evidence-based practice also contributed to the thinking behind the East Riding project: two national pilot sites in England, one at Leicester Royal Infirmary and at Kings Healthcare in London, and two health authority projects in Oxford and Sheffield. Also, the NHS-supported GRiPP[9] and Framework for Appropriate Care Throughout Sheffield (FACTS)[12] programmes both emphasised multidisciplinary approaches and change management skills, concentrating on motivation of staff and the identification of key local professionals. These two projects also attempted to take account of patients' views and behaviour. They thus shared common purpose with the East Riding initiative and, importantly, both were viewed in the NHS as successfully having achieved change in clinical practice.

The success criteria derived for the guidelines project proved strikingly similar to that of the Business Process Re-engineering project at Leicester Royal Infirmary, coincidentally strengthening the belief that the implementation of guidelines may critically rest on changing the culture and behaviour both of organisations and of individuals. At Leicester, an early quality improvement initiative had led to the introduction of a single visit neurology clinic. From this had grown a redesign programme for hospital services using business process re-engineering techniques, which are defined as:[13]

the fundamental rethinking and radical redesign of business processes to achieve dramatic improvements in critical, contemporary measures of performance, such as cost, quality, service and speed.

Applied by the Leicester Royal Infirmary, the working definition of re-engineering became 'the fundamental rethinking and radical redesign of an entire hospital system, including:

- healthcare processes
- jobs
- organisational structure
- management
- culture'.

Similarly, the working definition for the East Riding guidelines project became:

the radical design of an evidence-based healthcare system across the primary/secondary care sectors at both provider and purchaser level,

impacting particularly on healthcare process and culture (*see* Box 9.2).

Box 9.2: What is business process re-engineering?

Business process re-engineering is a concept used widely within industry and commerce which can be adapted and applied to healthcare to modernise and continuously improve the quality of our service.

Throughout the business of assessing health need, commissioning and delivering health services run several different processes. Those that are essential for the delivery of needs assessment, commissioning and delivering healthcare have been termed 'core business processes'.

Many health core processes have remained unchanged for years although there have been changes in staff and skilling and immense advances in technology.

With the patient at the heart of this methodology, services are systematically evaluated and, if necessary, redesigned. Ideally based on evidence of effective practice, the use of business process re-engineering allows for testing research findings by 'piloting' and 'prototyping' in real situations, such as hospital wards and general practice surgeries, before providing new ideas and concepts across hospitals or health authorities. Thus, research findings and theoretical concepts can be modified, taking on board the realities of day-to-day health service life. Used with care, the application of business process re-engineering to health services can achieve dramatic and sustainable results by eliminating the ineffectual and wasteful components of healthcare core processes.

Getting the project started

One of the first 'getting started' tasks was to establish an advisory group which pulled together key local stakeholders and was co-ordinated by a local general practitioner who was chair of the MAAG. This leadership and siting of the project was an important factor in its success, for while the project was able to establish its own identity it was also able to build on the work of the existing MAAG team, who had already created an environment of trust and respect among a broad multidisciplinary section of the local NHS community. Stakeholders in the advisory group included:

- Trust medical directors
- Continuing medical education tutors
- Local medical committee representatives
- Director of public health and public health consultants
- GP representatives
- MAAG members.

Nevertheless, although the configuration of the group represented a significant degree of local clinical ownership it soon became clear that other important multidisciplinary team members had been excluded (e.g. the group was very medically dominated). Consequently, some delay was experienced at the start of the project because time had to be spent identifying and recruiting senior nursing and management representatives (including information management and communications experts). Finally, a full-time project manager was then appointed who had both a clinical and a managerial background and had been trained as a change agent at Leicester Royal Infirmary.

New initiatives often succeed or fail not so much because of the technical aspects but as a result of the local environment. So, to prepare the ground for the East Riding initiative, the health authority:

- started to develop the evidence base for the index conditions
- spent time in managing the 'local politics'
- made links with several well-developed research and critical appraisal networks already helping practitioners to develop skills in evidence-based healthcare
- worked closely with the local educational strategy group, whose role it was to co-ordinate postgraduate education across all healthcare professionals within the area.

Who should do what?

Using methods developed at Leicester Royal Infirmary, a stakeholder analysis interview was completed for each clinical topic to identify the key individuals and organisations, to establish their possible position within the project and to use their ideas and concerns about guidelines to shape the project design. External experts in the clinical area were then interviewed and the content of these interviews recorded and incorporated in designing an external appraisal of the project.

Stakeholders and organisations had identified their initial priorities for guideline development in the analysis phase and decisions were made on which of these to select based on the amount of good quality evidence (clinical, managerial and economic) available in each clinical area. At this early stage three prototype areas for local clinical guideline development and implementation were selected as being (relatively) straightforward and where the majority of stakeholders agreed that these were priorities locally which would target areas of need. These were:

- acute low back pain management

- use of lumbo-sacral spine X-rays

- prescription of aspirin for post-myocardial infarct patients.

For each of these three areas there was reasonable evidence of effectiveness (or ineffectiveness) of therapy and, in the case of lumbar spine X-rays and the management of low back pain, evidence-based guidelines had already been developed nationally. In the third case, aspirin in the management of acute myocardial infarction, there was a wealth of evidence available but a national guideline did not exist at the time the project was commissioned.

Finding 'product champions'

Leaders for the implementation projects were chosen from among clinicians who were identified locally as being highly respected individuals, and who had a genuine interest in driving guideline implementation in their clinical area. Links with the local postgraduate medical school meant that senior academic staff could be involved on a regular basis (e.g. as 'project champions'). It also enabled joint working with academic colleagues to create evidence bases and to design organisational and educational systems, making good use of the expertise and information available locally. Performance measures and specific targets were developed for each potential guideline.

Bringing it all together

Once all of the information from this 'who and what' phase had been assembled and sorted into a logical sequence it was presented to the project steering group and other expert individuals. Facilitation of the process took place in the form of 'visioning workshops', where participants were encouraged to think outside of their normal sphere of expertise, to search for innovative and unconventional ideas which could be used to generate options for the next stage of the process – 'prototyping'.

The role of prototypes is to test the theoretical model in safe reality, therefore prototype sites usually include volunteers and enthusiasts and have a higher than usual chance of success, in turn rapidly generating a high level of respect and interest. For each clinical area several general practices volunteered to work together with the relevant hospital departments. Groups from the private sector also volunteered to act as prototype sites, working alongside NHS colleagues.

A 'visioning' workshop focused on each clinical area, bringing together multidisciplinary and multisectoral groups. Participants came from a variety of backgrounds including academic staff, primary and secondary care clinicians and healthcare professionals, local health authority, hospital and primary care managers and, importantly, consumers. The term 'visioning' was not used with the groups initially since jargon was identified as a potential problem at an early stage within the project's development. Many clinicians found this type of management jargon uncomfortable and too alien. In order to encourage maximum participation language was kept as familiar and straightforward as possible.

Highly respected senior colleagues, often from national bodies or international teams, but brought in because the local stakeholders had requested their presence, took part in the workshops. These individuals were active within small groups alongside local delegates and played a critical role in stimulating debate and introducing new ideas.

First steps in implementation

Mapping the evidence

Starting with a detailed, five-month long, development phase, the project used the rigorous approach of evidence-based healthcare as taught by the Oxford Critical Appraisal Skills Programme.[12]

The first part of this process was a detailed mapping exercise of all existing work on guidelines locally, nationally and internationally, for the three index conditions: back pain, lumbo-sacral spine X-ray and aspirin therapy in post-myocardial coronary heart disease. Simultaneously, published and unpublished literature was systematically searched, using graded evidence where possible, from four databases (HELMIS, PSYCHLIT, MEDLINE and Cochrane).

Proceedings from the workshops were circulated for comment to those who attended (and also those who were unable to attend), after which the draft guideline was modified in accordance with local consensus but without disputing the evidence base. This second draft was circulated for a two-month period of consultation to all those involved with the initial scoping process analysis (300 GPs and their teams, local hospital departments of cardiology, rheumatology, healthcare of the elderly, clinical audit and coronary care, and to the ambulance service).

The finalised guideline was disseminated as a package containing a short evidence-based bullet point version of the guideline, an audit proforma and a patient information sheet. An example of the 1996 short form of the lumbo-sacral X-ray guideline is shown in Box 9.3.

Box 9.3: The East Riding Guidelines Initiative (1996 short form)

Indications for lumbo-sacral spine X-ray in acute back pain

Back pain with neurological signs of cauda equina compression must be referred for neurological opinion.

X-ray required in:	*Age range (years)*
Children, especially painful scoliosis	< 18
Systemic signs, raised ESR, nocturnal pain	All
Disproportionate sacral distribution	All
Suspicion of metastases or osteoporotic collapse	65+
First episode 6 weeks plus duration	up to 18/65+
Recurrent episodes × 2+ in 6-month period	up to 18/65+
X-ray not required in:	
First episode	18–65

Baselining

Establishing an understanding of the 'where are we now' position was considered an important prerequisite for monitoring the impact of the East Riding initiative, since it would enable the measurement and assessment of any changes that might occur subsequent to the implementation of the guideline. Therefore, the first step was to explore practitioner opinion and practice in specific areas of the guideline (e.g. usage of lumbar spine X-ray), so providing a firm foundation against which to measure change by repeating the same processes six months after implementation. Audits of the three clinical areas were also planned, using performance measures derived from the evidence bases. For example, 'Was medication prescribed in accordance with the advice contained with the guideline and were services used in the way recommended by the guideline?' These initial audits took place retrospectively, examining records of clinical practice at least 12 months before the inception of the East Riding initiative (*see* Box 9.4 for an example).

Box 9.4: The lumbar spine X-ray guideline

Objective

The use of this guideline will result in a 50% reduction across the health authority area in the numbers of referrals for lumbar spine X-ray.

Approach

The guideline implementation process will involve all GP practices, acute and community hospitals (departments of radiology, orthopaedics, rheumatology, physiotherapy).

- Physiotherapists (private sector), osteopaths, chiropractors
- Community health councils, patient groups
- Private hospitals.

Baseline data collection

1 Referral rates by list size, clinical, etc., for the above groups.
2 Epidemiological data (e.g. Jarman score).
3 Survey of general practitioners' opinions on the role of radiology in patients with low back pain.

Guideline recommendations (*see* Box 9.3)

Anticipated outcome

1 Fall in referral rates at 3 months post-guideline implementation.

2 Identification of specific problems in areas of high referrals.

3 Redesign of referral system to eliminate inappropriate referral.

4 Introduction of educational interventions and support for inappropriate high referrers.

Benefits for patients

1 Reduction in radiation.

2 Elimination of unnecessary visits.

3 Shortened waiting time for other investigations.

Benefits for referrers and the radiology services

1 Increased positive yield therefore clinical intervention more effective.

2 Cost savings.

3 Faster access as a result of reduced usage.

Evaluation

Repeat audits planned at 6-monthly intervals.

Rolling out the programme to other clinical areas

Once the three prototype teams, working on back pain, lumbo-sacral spine X-ray and aspirin therapy, had created draft guidelines a substantial body of interest started to develop locally. A core group of 79 general practice teams (out of a possible 97) became actively involved, taking part in workshops, interviews, audits and specific problem-solving groups. In addition, volunteer pilot projects came forward from each of the four local hospitals, forming implementation teams to test the generic model in practice.

Eight more clinical areas were selected by a prioritisation process which involved interviewing senior health authority and hospital staff and primary care teams, an analysis of epidemiological data and existing local audits. Each area was agreed with the health authority. The intention was to pilot, modify and then roll out systematically each project across the whole sponsoring organisation. The eight proposed areas were:

- cardiopulmonary resuscitation skills for citizens (led by the local ambulance service)
- cardiac rehabilitation (led by the University of Hull)
- 24-hour emergency care (hospital and general practice)
- diabetes (acute trust, health authority and general practice)
- cancers (led by the local cancer centre)
- lipids therapy (health authority and all trusts and general practice)
- mental health – depression (community trust)
- discharge planning: fractured neck of femur (acute and community trusts)

Each team recruited by senior management within the hospitals, and the ambulance service and in primary care teams, consisted of experienced individuals with the ability to drive change and possessing skills ranging from leadership to data analysis. Support was provided by the East Riding guidelines team who would bring in training (e.g. critical appraisal skills programmes) or assist with the development of evidence bases and support service redesign. Care was taken to act in an advisory capacity only, since the programme was about creating the ability within organisations to design and deliver their own evidence-based healthcare.

Ensuring smooth progress

Four essential elements of the East Riding initiative were needed to lay the groundwork for success.

1 Communication.

2 Resources.

3 Quality assurance mechanisms.

4 User involvement.

Communication

A specific communication approach was developed to ensure that all hospitals and targeted clinical groups were aware of the project, including its potential implications for local services, and to facilitate the introduction and implementation of the guidelines into clinical practice. The objectives of the communications strategy were:

- to provide a clear and accurate picture of the guidelines development throughout the duration of the project
- to establish two-way communication with key stakeholders
- to facilitate the implementation of specific guidelines
- to enhance co-ordination of services between primary and secondary care.

Consumers, patients and potential patients, were included within the communications strategy, since part of the guidelines approach involved patient education. For instance, in the case of the lumbar spine X-ray guidelines, early investigation showed that some patients actually viewed radiological investigation as part of the treatment for low back pain. As a consequence, if patients were not offered an X-ray they had a tendency to be dissatisfied.

One of the patient education methods used was to arrange for GPs and implementation teams to take part in local radio programmes, followed by a programme of events for local consumers. Written material was published in local newspapers and patient leaflets, informing service users and members of the public about the risks of harm from radiation doses and the appropriate role played by radiology in the management of low back pain. The programme also targeted all local service providers and other departments within the health authority, with separate events for different audiences. Articles drawn from local and national publications were used to influence local opinion.

Resources

A belief held by the East Riding team was that all too often an expressed concern over lack of resources is sometimes used as an excuse not to do things, rather than as a stimulus to think of innovative solutions and different, less resource-intensive ways of working. For instance, much of the 'pump-priming' funds allocated to the two re-engineering national hospital pilot sites at Leicester and in London had been used to develop a strategic framework and practical tools, and to test in practical locations new solutions to old problems, rather than support infra-structure. In changing practice and culture, it is not always necessary to start from scratch. The two national hospital sites took high risks, as business process re-engineering can be a difficult and painful process. But then the information generated by pilot sites can be used by others to gain some of the benefits experienced without taking the same levels of risk themselves.

Thus, a key feature of the East Riding approach was to tap into existing resources by designing the programme as an integral part of daily working life. Designing the 'old' out of existence and introducing new evidence-based systems presents the opportunity for creating sustained change and preventing poor working practice.

Resources are always a challenge, however. Although a financial commitment was made by the health authority to supporting the guidelines initiative, it was not always possible to access all that was needed. Therefore, external resources (e.g. research monies and grants from the private health sector) were utilised to subsidise parts of the East Riding programme, particularly for training and to second staff to develop evidence bases. However, no more than 10% of the project was funded in this way.

Quality assurance mechanisms

Several quality checks were carried out as a routine part of the programme to ensure that the thinking and early model development was robust and likely to deliver the intended results. This quality cycle had three principal steps:

1 Challenging individuals, from within organisations attempting to achieve the change, are invited to short events along with others from outside (e.g. the NHS Executive or centres of good practice in the topic area).

2 Members of the project team present their findings at planned stages throughout the programme at these events.

3 This whole project team then reviews and critiques the findings. Comments are noted and researched and, if valid, the programme is modified.

User involvement

If guidelines are to be effective then they have to take account of evidence generated by the service users and members of the public. At the Leicester Royal Infirmary, for instance, the Patients' Council played a fundamental role in designing the programme and this approach fits with a specific NHS requirement to 'Give greater voice and influence to users of NHS services and their carers in their own care, the development and definition of standards set for NHS services locally and the development of NHS policy. . . '.[13]

Because the project workload was found to be mainly concerned with clinical problems, and of greatest prevalence in areas of high deprivation, two distinct methods of involving consumers were used. First, as a means of incorporating the views of groups already involved in local healthcare, it was decided to utilise existing mechanisms (e.g. community health councils and other public groups such as Rotary Clubs) to gain an understanding of the users' role in changing practice to a more evidence-based approach. The initiative sought to involve these groups routinely as stakeholders, in the same way as other professional groups. Second, a local company with expertise in consumer involvement in public sector organisations was engaged to target individuals from a defined geographical area, initially by letter. Representatives from the company then interviewed members of the public using predetermined sample criteria (e.g. members of patient pressure groups were excluded since it was considered important that the group should maintain neutrality as far as possible). The process resulted in the recruitment of a panel of 17 individuals, with ages ranging from 32 to 69 years (40% female). The panel was trained during an evening session, covering basic subjects such as confidentiality, the aims of the project and 'What are guidelines?', with time allowed for participants to express their hopes and concerns for the outcome of the work. This group became a 'citizens council', and began to take part in multidisciplinary workshops alongside clinicians and other healthcare professionals, helping to design and review evidence-based guidelines centred around care pathways.

In conclusion: has it made a difference?

Early signs of success started to appear nine months after the project started, with enthusiastic responses to the initiative from local clinical teams. Clinical audit based on evidence was built into the project design as an integral part of its implementation and to establish the programme's effectiveness more robustly a separate external assessment was undertaken.

Semi-structured interviews were undertaken to evaluate the impact of the East Riding Guidelines Initiative, and audit results provided the quantitive component. Following the implementation of the aspirin guideline there was a rise in compliance from a baseline of 57% to 72% within six months of receipt of the guideline. A number of the GPs commented that they had altered their referral patterns as a result of the acute back pain guideline, and many commented on the usefulness of using the guideline to inform patients on appropriate management of back pain.

Independent evaluation also indicated that the guidelines were being used by the health authority, local hospitals and general practices to business plan and to predict activity levels for many of the guideline topics.

Evidence from organisational change models, such as process re-engineering, suggests sustainable and significant quality improvement gains in clinical and other NHS services can be achieved. Experience in the East Riding project supports the view that it is possible to implement evidence-based practice using a multifaceted approach that includes a business process, although further research is required to explore the wider application of these models.

If this information on guideline implementation is to be transferred, enabling sites to adopt their own approaches, then aggressive marketing of existing models and practical help (using change agents among others) in applying quality tools will be essential. Exactly how this takes place is not yet clear but there is surely a role for a centrally supported body to draw together the evidence produced throughout the health and educational sectors to facilitate actively the process. The success of the Scottish Clinical Resource and Audit Group (CRAG) and the Northern Ireland CREST (Clinical Resource and Evaluation Support Team) suggests that this is a role which could also be played by the new English National Institute for Clinical Excellence (NICE).

References

1 National Health Service Executive Letter (1993) *115: Improving Clinical Effectiveness*. NHS Executive, London.
2 National Health Service Executive Letter (1994) *74: Improving the Effectiveness of the NHS*. NHS Executive, London.

3 National Health Service Executive Letter (1995) *68: Priorities and Planning Guidance for 1996/97*. NHS Executive, London.

4 Oxman AD, Thomson MA, Davis DA and Haynes RB (1995) No magic bullets: a systematic review of 102 trials of interventions to improve professional practice. *Canadian Medical Association Journal*, **153**: 1423–31.

5 Grimshaw J and Russell IT (1993) Effect of clinical guidelines on medical practice: a systematic review of rigorous evaluations. *Lancet*, **342**: 1317–22.

6 Grol R (1992) Implementing guidelines in general practice care. *Quality in Health Care*, **1**: 184–91.

7 Lomas J (1993). Making clinical policy explicit: legislative policy making and lessons for developing practice guidelines. *International Journal of Technology Assessment in Health Care*, **9**: 11–25.

8 Gilbert D, Dunnwig M and Gerrard A (1998) UK PACE projects. *Healthcare Quality*, **4**: 30–4.

9 Anglia and Oxford Regional Health Authority (1994) *Getting Research into Practice and Purchasing (GRiPP)*. NHS Executive, Oxford.

10 Royal College of General Practitioners (1995) *The Development and Implementation of Clinical Guidelines: Report of the Clinical Guidelines Working Group*. Report from Practice 26. RCGP, London.

11 Crombie I (1996) *The Pocket Guide to Critical Appraisal*. British Medical Journal Publishing, London.

12 Eve R, Golton I, Hodgkin P, Munro J and Musson G. (1997) *Occasional Paper 97/3. Learning from FACTS*. Scharr, Sheffield.

13 Department of Health (1996) *Local Voices*. HSMO, London.

10
Using guidelines to commission healthcare

Nicholas Hicks

All the available evidence suggests that guidelines do not implement themselves – systems are needed to support the implementation process. One important approach that has developed in the National Health Service is through the commissioning of healthcare, a model which healthcare purchasers have used in a number of other countries, particularly in North America. This chapter reviews some of the successes and the difficulty in commissioning using guidelines as the basis for improving patient care. It examines some of the evidence of the effectiveness of health improvement commissioning and draws on a number of successful approaches to demonstrate how progress might be made locally.

Introduction

Healthcare systems around the world face a number of very similar problems. One response to these problems is to separate the responsibilities for planning and paying for healthcare from responsibility for providing healthcare. Organisations that plan and pay for healthcare for defined populations are referred to as 'healthcare commissioners'. Their make-up and background may be very different, for they may be insurance companies, health authorities and health boards, health maintenance organisations or groups of general practitioners. But they all have a similar interest in ensuring the provision of effective, efficiently delivered healthcare. This chapter considers how guidelines can be used by commissioners to tackle some of the major issues faced by healthcare systems around the world.

The context

In recent decades it has become apparent that many of the major problems of the UK National Health Service are shared with healthcare systems across the developed world. In every developed country, where data have been sought, healthcare systems demonstrate:

- widespread variations in the rates of delivery of healthcare, both within and between countries

- escalating healthcare costs and an inability of even the richest countries to pay for all the healthcare demanded by the public and by the healthcare professions

- uncertain links between investment in healthcare, the delivery of healthcare and improvements in the health of individuals and populations

- the apparently incomplete, inaccurate and slow reflection of valid, relevant research findings in clinical practice.

The typical reaction to this set of issues among those that pay for and use health services has been to demand greater accountability from those that provide health services. In particular, there is an increasing expectation on the providers of care that they should be able to demonstrate the *value of* healthcare by better relating improvements in health to the consumption of resources.

In recent years, the problems have been so great that many countries (including the UK, US, New Zealand, France and Sweden) have reviewed and in some cases fundamentally reformed their arrangements for funding and delivering healthcare. However, given that the problems prompting healthcare reform are seen in privately funded healthcare systems, insurance-based systems, tax-funded healthcare systems, in market-based systems, and planned healthcare systems, there is a growing realisation that large-scale 'macro' structural healthcare reform is unlikely to solve the major effectiveness, cost-effectiveness and quality issues.

A very different approach to tackling the issues identified above comes from considering the pattern of healthcare, the allocation of healthcare resources, and the effectiveness of a healthcare system as the products of many hundreds of thousands of individual clinical decisions. From this 'micro' perspective, the problems of healthcare systems, such as variations in clinical practice and the imperfect use of valid research findings, become symptoms of imperfect clinical decision making rather than symptoms of imperfect health system design. This prompts the simple but important question: 'How can a healthcare system support and promote high quality clinical decision taking?' or alternatively 'How can a healthcare system promote clinical effectiveness?' Surprisingly, these are relatively new questions in healthcare policy circles.

Answering these questions has stimulated much study of the determinants of clinical decision making and clinical behaviour and of the link between research and clinical practice. Results suggest that judicious use of clinical practice guidelines and application of the principles advocated by the 'evidence-based healthcare' movement can improve the quality of clinical practice. Policy makers and practitioners are now beginning to explore how the theory of effective guideline development and use, and the principles of evidence-based healthcare can best be applied in practice in various healthcare systems.

Commissioning healthcare

A number of countries, including the UK, have separated the organisational responsibilities for population planning and the purchasing of healthcare from the provision of health services. In the UK, commissioners of healthcare receive a sum of money to buy healthcare for a defined population. They are expected to assess the needs of their population and then to purchase healthcare to meet those needs from one or more providers of health services. These tasks are now shared between general practice and health authorities/boards, although the latter initially held the principal responsibility.

Understanding how guidelines might help in commissioning healthcare requires an understanding both of the types of decisions that a healthcare commissioner takes and of the types of decision in which they have a legitimate interest. The variety of tasks that a commissioner might be involved in is illustrated by the aims and objectives identified in 1990 by Bristol and Weston Health Authority, in the early years of the internal market in the NHS (*see* Box 10.1).

Box 10.1: Commissioning healthcare: aims and objectives

The Authority's overall goal is: 'To deploy available resources to optimise the health of the population of Bristol and Weston District' by:

1 reducing the burden of existing disease

2 preventing new disease

3 promoting actions and values that contribute to good health.

Specific objectives

The Authority will aim to:

1 measure the health of the resident population and identify the determinants of the population's health

2 identify services that are effective in improving health and relate them to the health of the resident population

3 obtain a full range of efficient, effective and appropriate services for its residents within the limits of resources available

4 set and monitor standards for health services and targets for improving the health of the resident population

5 encourage residents and others to participate in making choices about the delivery of effective health services

6 inform the resident population of influences on their health and of actions that they or others might take to improve it

7 ensure that appropriate services are delivered unhindered by ability to pay, geographical location, gender, ethnic background or social class.

Commissioning and clinical effectiveness

In 1990, Bristol and Weston Health Authority wrote explicitly of 'obtaining a full range of effective services . . .'. It is implicit in what they wrote that they wanted to direct their resources into services that were *effective* in: (a) reducing the burden of existing disease, (b) preventing new disease and (c) promoting actions and values that contribute to good health. This emphasis on effectiveness has subsequently become a high priority for the entire NHS, as it has for most developed health services. As a consequence, the NHS Executive now expects that throughout the NHS 'decisions should be formulated on the basis of appropriate evidence about clinical effectiveness'.[1,2] This exhortation applies as much to commissioners as it does to providers of healthcare.

If it is accepted that the major issues of healthcare are not likely to be addressed solely by macro-structural change, then commissioners must also concern themselves with the clinical and financial consequences of the individual clinical decisions taken in the services that they seek to have provided. Thus, the sorts of practices and decisions that a commissioner will seek to promote include:

- the identification and withdrawal of resources from services that are ineffective, for example, dilatation and curettage in young women for the treatment of abnormal uterine bleeding, lumbar spine X-ray in the investigation of low back pain (*see also* Chapters 2 and 9)

- the identification and promotion of the widespread use of care that both improves health and saves money, for example, aspirin and beta blockers to prevent further cardiovascular events in people who have had a myocardial infarction

- the identification of treatments of equal effectiveness so that, among treatments of equal effectiveness, cheaper treatments can be substituted for more expensive forms of care, for example, substitute lansoprazole for omeprazole in the treatment of dyspepsia

- the identification and removal of inefficient practices, waste and duplication in the delivery of healthcare, for example, promotion of electronic rather than paper communication and the elimination of referrals to hospital out-patients for the sole purpose of obtaining an investigation that could be ordered directly from primary care

- in the light of information about the cost-effectiveness of services, the replacement of less cost-effective care with more cost-effective care.

Each of these is an example of the products of good commissioning. Some of these may be decisions that are taken by commissioners themselves, but more frequently these will be the sorts of decisions that commissioners will want to promote among those it commissions to provide care. Commissioning healthcare is therefore just as much about influencing and improving the quality of clinical practice as it is about making investment and health policy decisions.

Getting research into practice: the role of guidelines

If commissioners aim to improve the cost-effectiveness of the care they commission they need to understand how to influence clinical practice. Understanding how research finds its way into practice is one way of learning about the factors that determine clinical behaviour change.

In recent years, the processes by which research findings flow into clinical practice have been studied by researchers from various disciplines including social and behavioural scientists, health services researchers, advertisers, and epidemiologists. Each of these disciplines confirms that the process by which research findings find their way into clinical practice is often complex and convoluted. However, Lomas has described[3] how the findings of each discipline are consistent with a model in which this flow can be thought of in three separate stages (*see* Figure 10.1):

1 diffusion

2 dissemination

3 implementation.

Diffusion is the passive spread of research findings. It includes the publication of research findings in peer-reviewed journals. Given that there are more than 20 000 biomedical journals in print[4] it is not surprising that it is almost impossible for any practitioner to identify, obtain and read all the articles that might be relevant to their practice, let alone appraise the articles and assimilate the findings in their practice. The implication is that it is naïve to believe that the mere publication of research findings will be sufficient to stimulate a universal change in practice. Yet, until recently, many people have assumed that publication is all that is required to get research into practice.

As the limitations of publication as a means of influencing behaviour have become better recognised, people have begun to take active steps to distribute research findings. Typically, groups of experts and/or enthusiasts seek to distil the scientifically valid and ethically defensible messages from the literature, present them in an easy-to-read format and distribute these messages to relevant practitioners. Guidelines and the guideline movement can be thought of as part of a dissemination process.

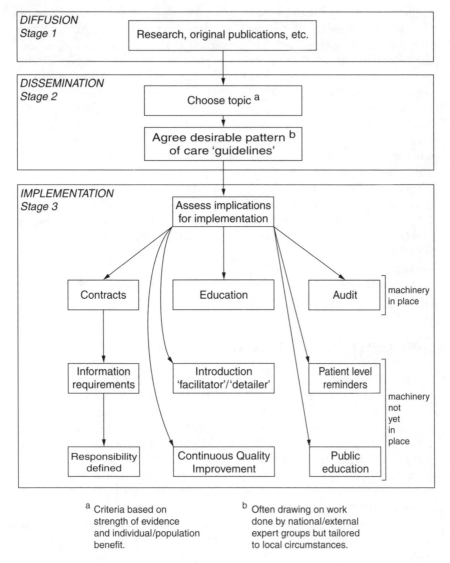

Figure 10.1 Getting research into practice.[3]

However, guideline producers and sponsors have often been disappointed at the lack of impact produced by their guidelines. In practice, even the best guidelines are often ignored, lost, thrown away, or simply not to hand when the information they contain might be of use to a practitioner.

There are many different ways in which professional practice can be influenced.[5] Methods that have been demonstrated to change practice include audit and feedback of performance,[6] education,[7] prompts and reminders delivered during the consultation,[8] opinions expressed by respected individuals and institutions,[9] relevant incentives and sanctions (which need not only be financial), one-to-one meetings (e.g. visits from pharmaceutical company representatives)[10] and changing patients' views of what to expect from healthcare. Encouragingly, where guidelines are supported by a planned process of implementation, there is good evidence that clinical practice can be changed so that care more closely reflects research findings.

These are important lessons for commissioners if they are to use guidelines in commissioning care successfully. Another important lesson, emphasised in other chapters in this book, is the importance of guidelines being 'owned' by those affected by their contents. If guidelines are to be effective in commissioning this has major implications for the way in which commissioners make their decisions. There is some evidence they are most likely to change clinical practice if they involve clinicians in their decision-making processes.[11]

'Top-down' and 'bottom-up' commissioning

When the internal market was introduced into the NHS, many people rather naïvely believed that written contracts between commissioner and provider would be an effective way of influencing clinical practice. Experience and experiment have demonstrated otherwise. For example, in one study designed to explore the potential of contracting to change professional behaviour, interviews with clinicians suggested that clinical practice was not influenced by clauses written into contracts when: (a) contracts were drawn up by people whose medical judgement clinicians did not respect (i.e. managers), (b) the documents were not read by clinicians (i.e. contracts) and (c) clinicians were excluded from the process of contract drafting. By contrast, clinicians saw the main determinants of their behaviour as their beliefs about what was in the best interest of each individual patient. Furthermore, these beliefs were influenced by their interpretation of the scientific literature and by the opinions of individuals and organisations that they respected.

Gradually, a more sophisticated way of conceptualising commissioning as a complex set of very different processes is emerging. At one end of a spectrum is a 'top-down' approach to commissioning which is most applicable for major public health and healthcare issues. At the other end of the spectrum is a 'bottom-up' approach to commissioning in which the commissioner fosters an environment in which the most appropriate clinical decisions are taken. Both of these approaches and the role of guidelines are outlined here.

'Top-down' commissioning can be thought of as a four-stage process that is very similar to the active process of translating research into practice described above. The four steps which form the backbone of the commissioning process (*see* Figure 10.2) are:

1 strategy formulation

2 programme specific policy development

3 implementation

4 monitoring.

I Strategy formulation

Every NHS healthcare commissioner, whether health authority, primary care group or fundholder, is subject to many influences and constraints. These include government policy, professional and expert advice, public opinion, local assessments of the health and healthcare needs of the population, and the financial position. Increasingly, therefore, commissioners are finding that dealing with these multiple pressures is only possible if they have identified and formulated a set of general principles, and agreed a general sense of direction. Such a set of principles and sense of direction is usually referred to as a strategy.

2 Programme specific policy

The next step is to break the task of commissioning a comprehensive range of healthcare services into manageable and clinically meaningful topics. Typically, these relate either to services for specific diseases (e.g. coronary heart disease), or to services for particular patient/client groups (e.g. people with learning disabilities). These sets of services are sometimes referred to as 'programmes of care' and health improvement programmes are an example of this approach. For each of these topics, a large commissioning agency, such as a health authority or health board, has the opportunity to act as ringmaster and bring together all the relevant stakeholders.

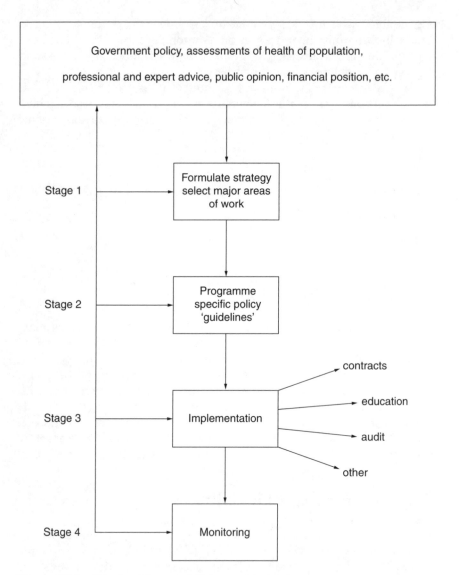

Figure 10.2 The backbone of the commissioning process.

For example, if the topic under discussion was the care of people with coronary heart disease, relevant stakeholders would include cardiologists, general physicians, geriatricians, cardiac surgeons, general practitioners, epidemiologists, rehabilitation staff, health promoters, and patients and their representatives. The purpose of bringing the groups together would be to debate and decide the optimal local pattern of care for people with heart disease. This agreement should be based upon an understanding of the incidence and prevalence of disease, valid and relevant evidence about the effectiveness and cost-effectiveness of different interventions, and the existing pattern of health services. This should lead to a shared understanding of how and where changes in services are needed and this shared understanding can be recorded in various forms. In the NHS, the most managerially familiar format of such an agreement has been the 'service specification', often structured as one or more clinical practice guidelines, superseded by the NHS frameworks.

If locally agreed practice change is recorded in guidelines, then guidelines have the potential to be the heart of commissioning. The guidelines can be referred to in, or become an integral part of, the agreements between commissioner and provider. But the theory of how research flows into practice (*see* above and Chapter 8) suggests that just agreeing service specifications/clinical guidelines is unlikely to produce change. The agreed guidelines need to be turned into practice through an active and planned implementation programme.

3 Implementation

Once there is a shared understanding and agreement about what changes in practice are required it becomes possible to develop a planned programme of implementation. The key is to make use of all the relevant effective methods of implementation. These include clinical audit and feedback, education, computer prompts, the provision of patient and public information, facilitation and appropriate use of local agreements on service provision (once called contracting!).

The contract had two main roles: (1) to help move necessary resources to where they are most needed, and (2) to document the various actions that different parties have agreed to and identify who is responsible for doing what and by when. These functions will still be needed in local agreements. For example, if it is agreed that general practitioners should have better access to echocardiography to guide their management of people who are suspected of having heart failure, then the contract can specify the relevant changes in provision of echocardiography. And it can record the date by which the new service should be in place, the criteria for access and for demonstrating that the service is being provided to the expected standards. Thus, although the contract alone is not effective at producing change, it does have a role to play in supporting and maintaining change.

4 Monitoring

Once there are explicit statements, whether as guidelines or as service specifications about the nature and quality of care that are linked to evidence and supported by all relevant parties, a number of other benefits of using guidelines become apparent. In particular it becomes possible to:

- derive clinically relevant measures of the quality of care
- identify particular processes where quality of care is imperfect
- take action to correct deficiencies in care
- improve the ability of health services to account for their use of resources.

The implication is that if guidelines are to be used in commissioning, then the whole process of commissioning of healthcare has to be driven by the process of agreeing and negotiating optimal patterns of care for particular diseases and patient/client groups.

An example of 'top-down' commissioning with guidelines

Tables 10.1 and 10.2 show how Oxfordshire Health Authority has incorporated evidence into its commissioning of care for coronary heart disease (CHD). The examples shown relate to services for the prevention of CHD:

- the evidence about effectiveness was discussed and agreed with relevant providers
- an ideal pattern of care for Oxfordshire as a whole was then described and agreed (*see* Table 10.1)
- the contribution of individual providers was summarised
- markers of progress towards the ideal pattern of care identified (*see* Table 10.2)
- the people who were responsible for ensuring that particular information was collected and presented were identified
- dates for completion of specific tasks were identified.

Table 10.1: Oxfordshire Community Health Trust: care programme for CHD

Oxfordshire Health Promotion Unit

1 The services provided should reflect an equal balance of provision for the three major groups of risk factors. These are:
- smoking
- poor diet and obesity
- low levels of activity and high levels of stress.

2 Oxfordshire Health Promotion should develop a more prominent role in lobbying for political changes which could have a significant impact on risk factors. Focus areas are:
- taxation and advertising of tobacco products
- subsidised healthy foods.
- labelling of foods with nutritional information.

Services intended to reduce the incidence of smoking

1 Development of requirements and recommendations in *Health at Work in the NHS* via the hospital's health promotion co-ordinator.

2 Collaborate with school nurses to report on and evaluate current stop-smoking activity in schools.

3 Identify opportunities to work with primary healthcare teams (PHCTs) to develop a common approach to smoking in pregnancy and early parenthood, and to link this with dietary advice.

Services to increase levels of physical activity and reduce stress

1 The services should reflect the national 'More People More Active' campaign.

2 Identify areas to work with the physical education advisory teacher and school health nurses to evaluate current provision for activity in local schools, both within and apart from the National Curriculum, in order to identify areas of underprovision.

Services to improve diet and reduce incidence of obesity

1 All healthy eating advice should be drawn from evidence based nationally promoted documents such as the COMA report *Nutritional Aspects of Cardiovascular Disease* or the BGH *Balance of Good Health*.

2 Identify areas to collaborate with the community nutrition and dietetic team.

Table 10.2: Oxford Community Health Trust: Monitoring of the care programme contract for CHD

The care programme specifies a complex number of services in order to be as complete as possible. It would not be feasible for all these services to be monitored, and so a limited number of *quality indicators* should be agreed, which if monitored are most likely to reflect the working of the care programme.

It has to be emphasised that in the care programme approach, the use of 'contract monitoring' is to *facilitate discussion on the current restrictions and different approaches to improving practice.* It has been demonstrated that for clinical teams to be involved in self-audit, there are important educational benefits. It is hoped that information resulting from audits will inform on the actual problems that hinder the practice of evidence-based medicine. There will be *no penalties* for failure to meet targets. Suggested quality indicators are shown below.

Agency	Quality indicator	Quality monitoring method	Required by:
Oxfordshire Health Promotion Unit (HPU)	The HPU should collaborate with school nurses and dieticians and, when relevant, community midwives, to begin to develop a strategic approach to health promotion activity in schools	To write a report on current health promotion activity in schools in collaboration with school nurses	September 1996
Community Nutrition and Dietetics	There should be collaboration between dieticians and representatives of community midwives to develop a common approach to diet in pregnancy and early childhood	To write a brief report on the progress of collaborative work with the PHCTs community teams and community midwives on diet in pregnancy and early childhood	September 1996
Family Planning Services		No monitoring required	
School Health and Community Paediatric Service	The HPU should collaborate with school nurses and dieticians and, when relevant, community midwives, to begin to develop a strategic approach to health promotion activity in schools	To contribute to the report to be drawn up by the Health Promotion Unit	September 1996
	Health promotion training needs for school health nurses should be identified, and these needs met where possible by the HPU	To produce list of Health Promotion training opportunities taken by school health nurses	December 1996

Each of these documents became part of the contract between the health authority commissioners and the relevant provider of care. However, although the guidelines have become part of a contract, no one felt that they had unreasonable tasks imposed on them. The process of reviewing evidence had ensured that each part of the NHS involved in the prevention and treatment of CHD in Oxfordshire is working to a common agenda. Subsequently, this style of commissioning has been shown to be associated with high quality clinical practice.

'Bottom-up' commissioning of healthcare

It is a major undertaking to attempt to improve a complex area of healthcare. No commissioner will be able to tackle more than a handful of topics simultaneously. Furthermore, even if major topics such as ischaemic heart disease, depression and leading cancers, were dealt with by top-down commissioning this would not address the vast majority of clinical decisions that have to made every day, yet commissioners, patients and providers will all want to ensure that the principles of evidence-based healthcare are applied as widely as possible.

In undertaking this challenging task it is clear that commissioners are never going to know the detail of all the decisions taken by providers that commit their resources. They have to trust providers to make the decisions as wisely as possible. But they can work to promote high quality decision making and to ensure that the staff from whom they commission care work in environments that help them make best use of evidence through 'bottom-up' commissioning. This means promoting the following issues.

Commitment

This involves commissions working to ensure that there is a commitment and culture from those who provide services to make best use of information. Commissioners can help to promote such a culture by raising it with senior staff (both clinical and managerial) and with governing bodies of provider organisations. This function will be supported by new initiatives to ensure clinical governance in hospitals and in general practice.

Relevant skills

If decisions that affect the care of patients are to be taken with due weight afforded to all relevant, valid information then those who take decisions must have relevant skills such as: (a) knowing how to turn practical problems into well-structured, answerable questions, (b) knowing how to find and make sense of evidence (perhaps as evidence-based guidelines), and (c) knowing how to act on the evidence.

Timely access to relevant information

This means ensuring that provider staff whose decisions affect the care of patients have access to appropriate information software and hardware and that they know how to use it. It also means that they know about, and have access to, the most appropriate information sources. Again, evidence-based guidelines can be important.

Appropriate organisation of work

Commissioners should also seek to ensure that those from whom they buy their care are well managed, and that staff time and work are structured in such a way that people can use the skills and information sources outlined above. In many cases, this may mean a major reconsideration of the way staff time is used. For example, a primary care team cannot make a decision about how they will manage as a team, even the common conditions such as diabetes or hypertension, if there is no forum for the team to meet and agree a course of action. Once a process is in place for making decisions, then further attention has to be given to ensuring and demonstrating that the decisions are turned into practice. One simple step that a commissioner can take is to ensure that all those from whom it commissions care have a credible approach to improving the quality of care that they offer which is presented to the governing body of the commissioning organisation. Increasingly, evidence-based guidelines are likely to have a prominent role in provider's quality improvement strategies.

In summary, in bottom-up commissioning, each provider is expected to be able to describe the processes of quality assurance and quality improvement they use. Guidelines are likely to be an important component of providers' processes for improving care. Effective commissioning requires commissioners to know about the validity and relevance of the guidelines in use in the services they commission, and the extent to which they are followed in practice.

Practical issues

This chapter has argued that there are many similarities between the process of commissioning healthcare and the process by which research findings are translated into practice. It has also argued that guideline development and implementation can be central to the process of commissioning care provided that those providing services are fully involved in agreeing the content of relevant guidelines.

Earlier chapters in this book describe important attributes of guideline development and implementation that are associated with the successful use of guidelines in promoting high standards of clinical practice. The lessons of each chapter are relevant to the use of guidelines in commissioning. For guidelines should be seen as tools to be used to support and not dictate clinical practice; those developing guidelines should understand (or have access to people who understand) the strength of inference that can be drawn from particular pieces of evidence; if, as will often be the case, local programmes of care are based on guidelines developed elsewhere, there should be skills available locally to appraise the validity and relevance of the externally developed guidelines; and once a local pattern of care is agreed, it should be understood that practice is most likely to change if multiple methods of implementation are used to support the guidelines.

Conclusion: the commissioner's agenda

It is a major undertaking to address a complex area of healthcare. As no commissioner will be able to tackle more than a handful of topics simultaneously, commissioners will have to choose which topics are priorities for the very active style of commissioning described in this chapter. This implies that they have a mechanism for setting priorities – another difficult task.

There can be many stakeholders to involve and considerable amounts of evidence to consider. Good communication and sound project management are required if the whole process is not to dissolve into confusion, uncertainty and falsely raised expectations. Well-developed social skills and a very visible commitment to the interests of patients and the population are required by commissioners if they are to earn and keep the trust and respect of the diverse groups of people with whom they will have to work. This is particularly important as many groups will start by fearing that a commissioner's main interest is in saving money.

Until recently, the NHS commissioners' timetables have been dominated by the annual contracting round. During this process they have gradually learned that commissioning comprises a complex pattern of activities (bringing people together, developing a shared understanding of the relevant, valid evidence, agreeing necessary changes in healthcare delivery, implementing those changes and monitoring the impact of those changes) which often takes several years to complete. Tenacity is thus an important characteristic for commissioners if they are to stimulate lasting improvement in the quality of care.

A number of skills are required by commissioners if services are to be commissioned in the way that has been outlined in this chapter. This has relevance for the recruitment and training of commissioning staff. Relevant skills include the ability to turn problems into answerable questions, knowledge of how to find and interpret evidence, knowledge of how to appraise and adapt guidelines and, crucially, the ability to use guidelines to change clinical practice. Some of these skills remain in relatively short supply in the NHS, although a number of training programmes and courses, such as the critical appraisal skills projects, have evolved to address these needs.

Commissioning care might be a less daunting task if the NHS had access to a library of well-constructed, appraised, summarised guidelines that could be used as starting points for local modification. Access to such material could substantially reduce the number of times different local groups have to find, appraise and act on the same body of evidence (*see* Chapter 6). Currently, not only is there a shortage of high quality guidelines, but there is also no easy way for identifying and retrieving those that do exist. Filling this gap should be a priority for the NHS, although some of the research-funded libraries and the AHCPR Guidelines Clearing House may offer new and interesting alternatives.

A recurring message in this and other chapters is that there are many different ways of influencing clinical practice and that the greatest change is likely to come about when mutually consistent and reinforcing messages are received by practitioners and the public from a variety of different sources. Some methods for changing practice are already embedded within the NHS, for example, clinical audit, education and contracting. But there are other effective methods of changing practice that are not so systematically available, for example, computerised practice prompts, facilitation, and patient/public education. Commissioners will need to pay greater attention to ensuring that they are aware of and use effective means of changing clinical practice.

They might also want to consider which methods of implementation are not well catered for in their localities and what they might do to improve things. For example, is there a satisfactory information technology infrastructure to support access to and communication of relevant information? Do all the people who need to use computers have the necessary skills to do so? Are there adequate means of informing the public and patients about what to expect from the health service? It is important for commissioners to address issues such as these if they are to have any realistic hope that the decisions they take will be implemented.

Currently, where effective practice change methods are available, it is rare for their agendas to be co-ordinated and their work to be mutually reinforcing. Learning how to co-ordinate such previously independent and unrelated activities as education, clinical audit and contracting will be another urgent and major challenge for commissioners,

Guidelines can be central to commissioning care. But if the full potential of commissioning and of clinical guidelines is to be realised, there are substantial implications for the skills required by commissioners, for the information commissioners require, and for the management and co-ordination of the multiple influences on professional practice. Commissioning care to improve quality is still a relatively new activity: there is much that has yet to be learned and achieved.

References

1   National Health Service Executive Letter (1995) *68: NHS Priorities and Planning Guidance for 1996/97*. NHS Executive, London.
2   National Health Service Executive Letter (1995) *105: Improving the Effectiveness of Clinical Services*. NHS Executive, London.
3   Lomas J (1993) Diffusion, dissemination and implementation – who should do what. *Annals of the New York Academy of Sciences*, **703**: 226–35.
4   Mulrow CD (1995) Rationale for systematic reviews. In: I Chalmers and DG Altman (eds) *Systematic reviews*. British Medical Journal Publishing, London.
5   Grecco PJ and Eisenberg JM (1993) Changing physicians' practices. *NEJM*, **329**: 1271–4.
6   Berwick DM and Coltin KL (1986) Feedback reduces test use in a health maintenance organisation. *JAMA*, **255**: 1450–4.

7 Davis DA, Thomson MA, Oxman AD and Haynes B (1995) Changing physician performance – a systematic review of the effect of continuing medical education strategies. *JAMA*, **274**: 700–5.

8 Stiemey WM, Hui SL and McDonald CJ (1986) Delayed feedback of physician performance versus immediate reminders to performing preventive care: effects on physician compliance. *Medical Care*, **24**: 659–74.

9 Lomas J, Enkin M, Anderson GM, Hannah WJ, Vayda E and Singer J (1991) Opinion leaders vs audit and feedback to implement practice guidelines: delivery after previous caesarean section. *JAMA*, **265**: 2202–7.

10 Avorn J and Soumerai SB (1983) Improving drug-therapy decisions through educational outreach: a randomised controlled trial of academically based 'detailing'. *NEJM*, **308**: 1457–63.

11 The North of England Study of Standards and Performance in General Practice (1992) Medical audit in general practice I: effects on doctors' clinical behaviour for common childhood conditions. *BMJ*, **304**: 1480–4.

11
Using guidelines in caring for patients

Francine Cheater and Richard Baker

One function of clinical guidelines is to assist decision making by patients. However, they are not commonly used in this way. In this chapter, features of guidelines that would be helpful to patients are discussed, including accessibility, format and content. Then decision making itself is considered in order to identify possible approaches to guideline development that would make them more useful as aids to patients' decision making.

Introduction

In caring for patients, guidelines may be used in several ways. They can be used by practitioners as foundations for the advice they offer patients. They might be used to provide patients with up-to-date summaries of research evidence. Guidelines could also be used in a more active way to provide context-specific information to aid decision making, with the patient taking a variable and perhaps predominant role. The ethical arguments for involving patients in decision making have been broadly classified as deontological (patients are autonomous and therefore have a right to information and involvement in decisions about their care) and consequentialist (providing information leads to particular desirable consequences).[1] In this chapter we do not firmly adopt one or other of these positions, but instead choose a middle position. While we believe that patients do have rights to involvement in decision making, the amount, type and method of achieving involvement should take into account the proven positive and negative effects of such involvement on outcomes.

We will first consider characteristics of guidelines that might enable them to be used with patients, taking note of their impact on the outcome of care and the involvement of patients in decisions. The accessibility of guidelines, their format and content, all influence the extent to which they can assist patient and practitioner decision making. Secondly, we will discuss how guidelines might be used more effectively with patients in the future, and we will draw on theories relevant to clinical decision making.

Guidelines as sources of information

Access

Just as practitioners need up-to-date information about research evidence, patients want access to reliable information about effective management.[2] The quantity and type of information to which an individual has access may be key to patient involvement.[3] Patients' needs for information will vary,[4] although there is plenty of evidence that most people want reliable information about their illness and its treatment. A fraction of the information patients may wish to be given during consultations is illustrated in Table 11.1, yet there is evidence that doctors and other practitioners consistently underestimate patients' desire for information.[2]

Patients who are given comprehensive information are generally more satisfied with their care, are less anxious and adhere more readily to treatment.[5] Other benefits of information-giving include better functional and physiological health outcomes,[6-8] shorter hospital stays and reduced drug usage.[8] A psychological interpretation of the benefits of information suggests that it enables patients to develop effective coping mechanisms, so reducing the stress associated with illness.[9] The explanations that individuals receive about their illness and treatment can affect their expectations of successful recovery, and also the extent to which they take appropriate action to contribute to their own improvement.[10]

Few systematically developed guidelines have adequately taken into account the views and preferences of patients. Despite the emphasis on involving patients or their representatives in the development of guidelines,[11] the production of patient versions of guidelines is not yet common practice in the UK, as happens in the US.[12] For each of the twenty or so national guidelines released through the Agency for Health

Table 11.1: Information patients may require at different stages of their healthcare

Stage	Example of type of information
Pre-diagnosis	What tests will I need? What are they for? How quickly can I have them? Do I need to prepare for my tests (e.g. fasting)? Can someone come with me? How long will they take? Will it be painful? How accurate is the test? When will I know the results?
Diagnosis and prognosis	How ill am I? Will I get better? Why did I get ill? Could I have prevented it?
Treatment/management	Is there a treatment? Will it work? Will I make a complete recovery? Is there an alternative? Which works best? What does the treatment involve? Will I be in pain? Are there any side-effects? Will my work/personal/social life be affected? What will happen to me if I do not have treatment? What are the experiences of other patients with my illness? Who is the expert in this field? Which hospital is best at treating my condition? Will I eventually be able to resume a normal life again? Will my illness recur?
Self-care/aftercare	Will I be on treatment when I go back home? Will I (my family) be taught how to look after myself? How do I get new supplies when these run out? Who do I contact if there is a problem? When can I go back to work? What benefits am I entitled to? When is my follow-up appointment?

Care Policy and Research (AHCPR), a patient version consisting of five to six pages, explaining the condition and the treatment options, has also been published. For some guidelines (e.g. the urinary incontinence guidelines), a caregiver guide has also been produced. The effects of providing patients with information in this format have not been extensively assessed, but public demand appears to be considerable. For example, the announcement on television and radio of the AHCPR incontinence guidelines prompted thousands of telephone calls and letters from the public requesting information.[13] Furthermore, information printed in two newspaper columns produced over 60 000 calls and thousands of letters.

Although in the UK, versions of guidelines for use by patients are comparatively uncommon, a number of initiatives are under way to provide patients with good quality information about the effectiveness of interventions based on available evidence. The Promoting Patient Choice programme, at the King's Fund Development Centre in the UK, is producing systematically developed information packages to support patient involvement for the following conditions: urinary incontinence, depression and anxiety in Asian women, childhood nocturnal enuresis, colorectal cancer, post-surgical pain and chronic inflammatory bowel disease. The College of Health in the UK is also undertaking several projects to develop and evaluate methods of informing patient choice. For example, booklets containing communication tools to assist patients in discussions about alternative treatments are being developed for depression or menorrhagia, based on the recommendations of clinical effectiveness bulletins for these two conditions.[14, 15] Another project is producing research-based patient leaflets to meet the information needs of those undergoing minimal access surgical procedures. The informed choice initiative has produced research-based leaflets about the effectiveness of options for care during stages of pregnancy and childbirth for women, as well as practitioners.[16]

These initiatives use methods, such as focus groups, together with reviews of research that describes people's experiences, to identify needs and priorities for information defined by patients or potential users of the service. This information is then combined with existing research evidence about the effective management of specific conditions by drawing on available guidelines, systematic reviews or other sources of evidence.

Information derived from guidelines, or other forms of evidence, needs to be made accessible before it can be used by patients. The most suitable approach will depend upon the intended audience, their language, literacy level and any disabilities that might make access to information difficult.[1] The mode of delivery will also be influential in determining access. The informed choice initiative[16] recommended that leaflets be 'prescribed' for pregnant women at the time information would be most relevant to them, rather than through passive dissemination (e.g. leaflets left on the reception desk at the out-patient clinic). However, access to information via health services potentially places practitioners in the role of gatekeepers to information. The alternative of distribution of information through consumer groups may introduce bias in favour of the motivated and advantaged. To address these difficulties, AHCPR guidelines are routinely publicised through the media of television, radio and newspapers which ensure wide coverage. It seems that to ensure equity of access, information needs to be provided in a variety of forms, although the relative effectiveness of different methods of delivery, for different patient groups, has still to be established.

Format

The format of guideline information will influence whether and how it is used. To date, systematically developed guidelines for practitioners have been presented as full versions that include all the supporting evidence as well as copies of shorter summaries for easy reference. Other formats include bulletins, research articles, audiotapes, videos, posters and electronic versions, including interactive media. However, little is known about practitioners' preferences for different formats, whether preferences vary according to discipline and setting, and whether some formats are more effective than others in facilitating use and assimilation of material. A study in the UK showed that when asked, community nurses preferred to receive information about clinically effective leg ulcer treatment in the form of interactive education.[17] The resulting information pack and audiotape produced significant improvements in nurses' knowledge in a controlled trial.

Similarly, we know little about the effect different guideline formats might have on whether, and how, practitioners might use information with patients during consultations. For example, would on-line interactive computer guidelines be more likely to facilitate discussion between practitioner and patient in a consultation than information provided in a booklet form or summary card? Our knowledge about how patients would prefer to receive information distilled from guidelines is even less. Patient versions of guidelines, leaflets and booklets have been the most common formats used so far. Patient information may be of variable quality and criteria for its appraisal have been suggested[18–20] (see Box 11.1). It has been shown that information that is poorly presented can deter patients from taking up services[21, 22] and may misguide, rather than inform them.

Box 11.1: Criteria for appraising patient information

Readability	Is it of relevance to patients?
Legibility	Is it based on good evidence?
Recall of information	Is it free from bias?
Compliance	Do patients have skills to use it?
Patient satisfaction[18]	Does it enhance choice?[19, 20]

The effectiveness of computerised reminder systems in modifying clinical performance is well established[23] but the most appropriate methods for using computers during consultations are unclear, especially when the conditions being considered are relatively unstructured. Attention is beginning to turn to this issue and at least one model has been proposed.[24] However, although evidence about the value of these systems has been available for some years, they have only been used in relatively limited fields of clinical practice, perhaps because they relate to the more structured aspects of care such as monitoring of anticoagulant medication or diagnosis of acute abdominal pain. In a study of the effect of a computerised prompting system on the performance of preventive health procedures in general practice, the number of procedures increased but the patients' contribution to consultations declined.[25] They spoke less, and presented fewer problems.

Methods of empowering patients by helping them to become more actively involved in the consultation have been evaluated to some extent. Patient-generated question lists have been shown to improve joint communication by helping patients organise their thoughts in advance of their consultation.[25, 26] Training patients to develop their question-asking skills increased their level of participation in consultations in the primary care setting[27] and improved patients' functional outcomes in ulcer clinics in hospital.[28] Research in general practice consultations has shown that patients who asked questions were between twice and twenty times more likely to receive relevant information than those who did not.[29] Patients who actively contribute in the consultation are more likely to receive the type of practical information needed to help them make decisions.[30] Information provided on audiotapes has been found to be effective in patients with cancer, teaching them to be more proactive in their interactions with doctors.[31] However, their use in patients with poor prognoses, who use denial as a coping mechanism, may be harmful.[32] This reinforces the point that interventions used to enhance patient information and participation in decisions about care, need to be tailored to the specific wishes and needs of the individual.

Interactive video disks used in advance of the medical consultation have also been developed to involve patients in decision making for conditions such as benign prostatic hyperplasia (BPH), back pain, hypertension and breast cancer in the Shared Decision Making Programme (SDMP) in the US[33] and for BPH and mild hypertension in the UK. In the SDMP, patients pursued their own line of questioning and at the end of viewing were supplied with a written copy of questions they had asked and answers, plus a review of treatment alternatives. Evaluation confirmed its popularity with patients, who found it easy to use and relevant to their needs. Routine referrals of men with BPH to view the video disk resulted in a fall in the demand for surgery in the first three years, and patients were satisfied with their decisions not to have surgery.[33]

Another promising development concerns the use of patient-mediated interventions, which have the potential to change practitioner behaviour by giving patients information about guideline recommendations. For example, in North America, reminders (letters or telephone calls) and/or educational interventions targeted at patients have been effective in the implementation of national guidelines for topics including preventive care,[34] immunisation programmes[35] and blood pressure screening.[36] As yet, the comparative costs and benefits of patient-mediated interventions with other implementation strategies is unknown.

Content

To date, decisions about topics for guidelines, how they are developed and what they will cover have largely been determined by interested practitioners, managers, academics and specialists in guideline methodology. Therefore, they may not necessarily address conditions of priority to patients. Furthermore, many patients, particularly older people, do not present with a single, clear-cut condition or diagnosis, yet guidelines usually address the care of a single clinical condition. Guidelines will reflect implicit or explicit assumptions, values and beliefs of members of the guideline group, regardless of how impartial the process of guideline development appears to be.[37] These values and beliefs may be quite distinct from those of patients (or practitioners involved in providing everyday care, see Chapter 5).

The extent to which published guidelines reflect the information needs of practitioners and patients in their day-to-day encounters is also relatively unknown. Evidence from randomised controlled trials (RCTs) may produce guideline recommendations based on findings that only relate to subgroups of patients and may, therefore, have limited relevance for practitioners in their own settings. Similarly, guidelines that place exclusive emphasis on the results of RCTs are unlikely to be helpful to patients as many interventions have not, and are never likely to be, subjected to this form of evaluation.

Practitioners and patients may value and understand the knowledge and recommendations presented in guidelines in different ways. Patients may be pressurised by practitioners' professional authority to accept, or conversely, reject guideline recommendations. Practitioners' beliefs and attitudes will also influence whether and how guideline recommendations are presented to patients and whether they are taken up. Similarly, failure to adhere to guidelines may be due to pressures exerted by patients on practitioners. The incorporation of patient preferences may lead to poor health outcomes, for example, when patients favour a course of action that practitioners believe is not in their best interests.[38] However, practitioners do not necessarily know what is in the best personal interests of the individual patient, although from a societal perspective, the benefits and costs of providing a particular treatment may be very clear. Patients may prefer a more costly alternative to an equally effective intervention or desire treatments which have been shown to be ineffective. This is illustrated by legal cases involving patients with complaints against their local health authorities or providers, when their wishes have been overruled by healthcare staff. At an individual patient level, moral reasoning may be a far more potent factor influencing decision making than the presentation of research evidence about the efficacy of various interventions.

Healthcare interventions may have multiple outcomes, for example, pain, disability, psychological, social and family consequences and financial costs. Patients need information about all possible outcomes for available interventions, if they are to make informed choices among the alternatives. The outcomes measured in research are often developed from a practitioner, rather than a patient, perspective.[39] An over-emphasis on the technical or physical elements of care in guidelines may obscure psychological and social costs and benefits that may be equally or more important to patients in making informed decisions. For example, women with early breast cancer may want to be actively involved in decisions about radical mastectomy versus lumpectomy because of the possible psychosocial consequences of mutilating surgery on post-operative quality of life. Although patient involvement in decision making does not necessarily improve psychological well-being, the quality of information-giving during the consultation can have an impact on outcome.[40]

Clinical benefits are usually easier to measure than psychological, social and other health-related quality of life outcomes, hence information about the benefits of non-clinical aspects of care is often limited. Although practitioners and patients may agree about the importance of certain outcomes, judgements about the importance of others will vary. Similarly, the decision for one patient need not be the same as that for a nearly identical patient due to differences in demographic characteristics, health status and nature of the medical decision. Practitioners and patients may also assume different levels of involvement in decision making, at specific stages of care. For example, Chewing and Sleuth[41] suggest that patients are less likely to want to collaborate in decisions about diagnostic tests than decisions about treatment. However, for antenatal or genetic screening, patients are likely to have a range of preferences for testing.

Information on long-term outcomes may also be absent. Aspects of care for which there are uncertainties about the benefits of interventions and possible outcomes should be made explicit in guidelines, otherwise patients may be reluctant to consider outcomes which may be important to them, but have uncertain probability of occurrence.[1] For example, patients with cancer of the prostate may prefer watchful waiting rather than surgery or radiotherapy as there is uncertainty about the benefits of treatment.[42] However, practitioners, particularly doctors responsible for determining treatment, may experience considerable discomfort in disclosing uncertainty about treatment outcomes in discussions with their patients.[43] Research into appropriate ways of communicating uncertainty to patients is in its infancy. Patients and practitioners may also experience difficulties making decisions about treatment options when required to make judgements about outcomes for which they have no experience. Eddy[44] suggests that patients are given examples within their own range of experiences, with which to compare particular outcomes. For example, discomfort associated with a particular procedure might be compared with having a tooth pulled.

Understanding patient and practitioner decision making

In order to consider how guidelines might be used more effectively in caring for patients, we need to understand how decisions are made in clinical practice. Evidence-based clinical decision making has been conceptualised in a simple model comprising three interrelated elements: (1) practitioner's clinical expertise, (2) patient preferences and (3) research evidence[45] (*see* Figure 11.1). In addition, the expertise which patients or their families bring with them to the consultation should also be included in this model For example, patients with long-term health problems such as diabetes, cystic fibrosis or rheumatoid arthritis, accumulate considerable expertise in the self-management of their conditions. This will influence their decision making and should, therefore, be made explicit in the discussion between patient and practitioner.

A recent definition of evidence-based practice used the term 'judicious use of current best evidence'[45] to emphasise the need to incorporate clinical expertise and the unique circumstances of the individual patient, as integral components of clinical decision making. Complex issues lie beneath this definition. It could be inferred that decision making itself is simple, and that practitioners and patients adopt a rational approach in which the provision of information is followed by a logical assessment of the alternatives and selection of a clear course of action. In reality, the interplay between the provision of information and patient preferences is an obscure process in which many factors are taken into account by the patient.

One line of enquiry into this process involves decision analysis using utility measurement methods such as standard gamble and time trade-off.[46] The use of these techniques in developing guidelines that promote

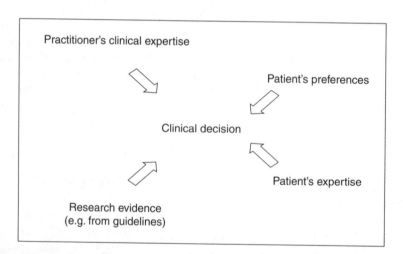

Figure 11.1 Factors influencing clinical decision making (from Haynes *et al.* 1996).[45]

patient involvement may initially appear attractive, but they are not without problems.[47] For example, the way in which options are framed may have a strong influence on the gamble taken (e.g. 90% survival vs. 10% mortality) and many people do not make decisions in this way.[38] Also, it is not clear that information presented in the form of probabilities of risk–benefit is meaningful to individual practitioners and patients. A study to assess methods of presenting data for treatment decisions on the management of hypertension indicated that most general practitioners had difficulty in interpreting the information.[48] The need to better understand how patients and practitioners make decisions, from a behavioural perspective, rather than relying solely on the traditional 'rational' model of decision making is clearly needed.

Theories of human behaviour may have more to offer than the traditional 'rational' model. For example, the theory of health locus of control[49] suggests that individuals differ in the extent to which they regard events as controllable by them. Those with an internal locus of control believe they have substantial control over their own health, while those with an external locus believe they have less control. Patients with an internal locus may be more likely to want information to help them make decisions about their care, but those with an external locus may find more information difficult to use and even disempowering. This may explain why some patients may not want to take part in decision making. For example, although the majority of patients with cancer want detailed information, the proportion that wish to be involved in decision making varies between 40 and 80%.[50–52]

Evidently, patients' preferences for participation in decision making lie along a continuum. At one extreme, some patients prefer to leave all decisions regarding treatment to their doctor or other member of the team (a passive role). Others prefer to share responsibility with their practitioner (a partnership role), but at the other extreme, some patients prefer to make the final choice about treatment (active role).[50] Clearly, the degree of patient involvement in decisions should depend on the wishes of the patient, which may be influenced by personal traits such as locus of control.

Several models have been developed in relation to patients' preventive health decisions. The health belief model[51] predicts that decision making will be influenced by four factors: (1) the patient's perception of personal susceptibility to the illness in question, (2) the severity of that illness, (3) the personal costs of making the decision, and (4) the benefits of the decision. This model has been criticised and studies of its ability to predict behaviour have had conflicting results, and other more complex models have been proposed, such as the theory of planned behaviour[53] or the health action process approach.[54]

Although these models have yet to be evaluated fully and generally relate to preventive health decisions, they do illustrate that the process by which individual patients make decisions is far from simple. The factors that influence practitioners in making decisions are also complex. In reaching a diagnosis, selecting an investigative procedure, offering information to the patient and recommending a therapeutic option, innumerable decisions must be made in quick succession. Attempts to understand the process of medical decision making have begun to recognise the influence of psychological and social factors.[55] The practitioner's perceptions of the patient's concerns have an impact on this process, for example, in prescribing decisions general practitioners have been shown to take social and other non-clinical factors into account.[56] The practitioner's own health beliefs may vary as much as the patient's, and may be a major influence on decision making.[57] Pre-existing beliefs about the nature, prevalence and incidence of clinical problems, the seriousness and treatability of the condition, experience accumulated during years of clinical practice, personal knowledge of the patient and personal values may all play a role.

One model of practitioners' decision making adopts a scientific perspective which makes the reasons for a decision transparent. The model argues that decisions could be improved by making more effective use of research evidence that takes into account the degree of certainty and patient preferences.[44] An alternative model suggests that professional knowledge is more than knowledge of the science of clinical practice, but also the daily application of that knowledge through reflecting on the outcomes of different actions.[58] In a synthesis of these alternatives, the cognitive continuum theory suggests that both the reflective and scientific approaches can be, and are, used by practitioners.[59] When tasks are relatively structured the scientific approach is used, when they are less structured a reflective or intuitive approach is adopted.

The committed empiricist may feel that there is little place for theories about the decision-making processes of patients and practitioners, and that all that is needed is a series of randomised controlled trials that evaluate the effectiveness of different methods of modifying decision making. Although the need for convincing empirical evidence is uncontestable, we also need ideas, or theories, to better understand the complicated processes involved in decision making, and to suggest possible interventions and postulate what their positive and negative effects might be. In particular, theories can indicate what outcome measures should be selected in trials, and what unwanted or adverse effects should be sought. For example, given the complex nature of decision making, there is a danger that guidelines could limit the opportunity of patients to choose the objectives of care. They might increase the role of decision making in relatively structured aspects of care and turn the attention of practitioners away from the less structured aspects. We need to be aware of, and investigate, these possibilities if we are to devise a 'best fit' between the interactions between patients and practitioners, and the methods used to inform the decisions they take together or individually.

Conclusion

The purpose of guidelines is to aid decision making by patients and practitioners, but as yet there is little experience of their use with patients. Extending their use with patients presents professionals with a difficult question – whether patient autonomy should take precedence, in which case guidelines should provide patients with all the necessary information for them to make their own decisions, if they so wish, or whether our prime responsibility is to guide our patients towards the decisions most likely to lead to the best clinical outcomes.

In this chapter we have shown that although attempts to develop and use guidelines with patients are relatively recent, there are many innovative developments, and many more ideas waiting to be evaluated. However, the approaches that have been adopted thus far have generally not taken into account the complex nature of decision making, except in a limited number of highly structured aspects of care. The risk is that guidelines, combined with over-zealous implementation, may dragoon patients into complying with clinical recommendations that do not fully accommodate their personal concerns.

Thus, we need more information about how communication between professionals and patients should proceed to ensure that patients are fully informed and may share decision making if they wish. However, a particular problem is that we do not yet fully understand the process by which patients and practitioners make decisions. There is a clear need for more detailed study of decision making in clinical practice, perhaps drawing on relevant behavioural theories. Nevertheless, some early experiments of shared decision making give rise to the hope that use of guidelines and sophisticated information technology may simultaneously improve patient information and involvement in decisions.

References

1 Entwistle VA, Sheldon TA, Sowden AJ and Watt IS (1996) Supporting consumer involvement in decision making: what constitutes quality in consumer health information? *International Journal for Quality in Health Care*, **8**: 425–37.

2 Coulter A (1996) *Developing Evidence-based Patient Information*. In: 'But will it work doctor?' Promoting and supporting patient choice by making evidence about the effectiveness of health care accessible to health service users. Report of a second 'But will it work doctor?' conference, 22–23 May, Northampton. (pp 30-32.)

3 Luker K, Beaver K, Leinster S, Owens G, Degner L and Sloan J (1995) The information needs of women newly diagnosed with breast cancer. *Journal of Advanced Nursing*, **22**: 134–41.

4 Cohen F and Lazurus RS (1982) Coping with the stresses of illness. In: GC Stone, F Cohen, NE Adler (eds) *Health Psychology*. Jossey-Bass, London.

5 Mosconi P, Meyerowitz B, Liberati M and Liberati A (1991) Disclosure of breast cancer diagnosis: patient and physician reports. GIVIO (Interdisciplinary Group for Cancer Care Evaluation, Italy). *Annals of Oncology*, **2**: 273–80.

6 Kaplan SH et al. (1989) Assessing the effects of physician–patient interactions on the outcomes of chronic disease. *Medical Care*, **27** (suppl): 110–27.

7 Schulman BA (1979) Active patient orientation and outcomes in hypertensive treatment. *Medical Care*, **17**: 267–81.

8 Hayward J (1975) *Information: A Prescription Against Pain*. Royal College of Nursing, London.

9 Janis IL and Rodin J (1982) Attribution, control and decision making: social psychology and health care. In: GC Stone, F Cohen and NE Adler (eds) *Health Psychology*. Jossey-Bass, London.

10 Wade B (1989) *A stoma is for life*. Scutari Press, London.

11 Duff L, Kelson M, Marriot S, McIntosh A, Brown S, Cape J, Marcus N and Traynor M (1996) Clinical guidelines: involving patients and users of services. *Journal of Clinical Effectiveness*, **1**: 104–11.

12 Van Amringe M and Shannon TE (1992) Awareness, assimilation and adoption: the challenge of effective dissemination and the first AHCPR-sponsored guidelines. *Quality Review Bulletin*, **18**: 397–404.

13 Colling J (1994) An update on the AHCPR guideline implementation. *Nurse Practitioner Forum*, **5**: 134–7.

14 National Health Service Centre for Reviews and Dissemination

(1993) *Effective Health Care. The Treatment of Depression in Primary Care.* NHS CRD, University of York.

15 National Health Service Centre for Reviews and Dissemination (1995) *Effective Health Care. The Management of Menorrhagia.* NHS CRD, University of York.

16 Rosser J, Watt IS and Entwhistle V (1996) Informed choice initiative: an example of reaching users with evidence-based information. *Journal of Clinical Effectiveness*, **1**: 143–5.

17 Luker K and Kendrick M (1995) Towards knowledge-based practice: an evaluation of a method of dissemination. *International Journal of Nursing Studies*, **32**: 59–67.

18 Arthur VAM (1995) Written patient information: a review of the literature. *Journal of Advance Nursing* **21**: 1081–6.

19 Hope T (1996) *Evidence-based patient choice and the doctor–patient relationship.* In: 'But will it work doctor?' Promoting and supporting patient choice by making evidence about the effectiveness of health care accessible to health service users. Report of a second 'But will it work, Doctor?' conference 22–23 May, Northampton. (pp 20–3.)

20 Gann B (1996) *Why share information with consumers?* In: 'But will it work, Doctor?' Promoting and supporting patient choice by making evidence about the effectiveness of healthcare accessible to health service users. Report of a second 'But will it work, Doctor?' conference 22–23 May, Northampton. (pp 38–43.)

21 Botha H, Manku-Scott T, Moledina F and Williams A (1993) Indirect discrimination and breast screening. *Ethnicity and Disease*, **3**: 195–8.

22 Goldsmith M (1992) Vaccine information pamphlets here, but some physicians react strongly. *JAMA*, **267**: 2005–7.

23 Shea S, DuMouchel W and Bahamonde L (1996) A meta-analysis of 16 randomized controlled trials to evaluate computer-based clinical reminder systems for preventive care in the ambulatory setting. *Journal of the American Medical Information Association*, **3**: 399–409.

24 Purves I (1996) Facing future challenges in general practice: a clinical method with computer support. *Family Practice*, **13**: 536–43.

25 Pringle M, Robins S and Brown G (1985) Computer assisted screening: effect on the patient and his consultation. *BMJ*, **290**: 1709–12.

26 Middleton J (1995) Asking patients to bring a list: feasibility study. *BMJ*, **311**: 34.

27 Roter D (1984) Patient question asking in patient–physician interaction. *Health Psychology*, **3**: 395–409.

28 Greenfield S, Kaplan S and Ware J (1985) Expanding patient involvement in care. *Annals of Internal Medicine*, **102**: 520–8.

29 Boreham P and Gibson D (1978) The informative process in primary medical consultations: a preliminary investigation. *Social Science and Medicine*, **12**: 409–16.

30 Tuckett D, Boulton M, Olson C and Williams A (1985) *Meetings between experts*. Tavistock, London.

31 Ford S, Fallowfield L, Hall A and Lewis S (1995) The influence of audiotapes on patient participation in the cancer consultation. *European Journal of Cancer*, **31A**: 2264–9.

32 McHugh P, Lewis S, Ford S, Newlands E, Rustin G, Coombes C, Smith D, O'Reilly S and Fallowfield L (1995) The efficacy of audiotapes in promoting psychological well-being in cancer patients: a randomised controlled trial. *British Journal of Cancer*, **71**: 388–92.

33 Kasper JF, Mulley AG and Wennberg JE (1992) Developing shared decision-making programs to improve the quality of health care. *Quality Review Bulletin*, **18**: 183–90.

34 Ornstein SM, Garr DR, Jenkins RG *et al.* (1991) Computer-generated physician and patient reminders. Tools to improve population adherence to selective patient services. *Journal of Family Practice*, **32**: 82–90.

35 Rosser WW, McDowell I and Newell C (1991) Use of reminders for preventive procedures in family medicine. *Canadian Medical Association Journal*, **145**: 807–14.

36 McDowell I, Newell C and Rosser W (1989) A randomised trial of computerised reminders for blood pressure screening in primary care. *Medical Care*, **27**: 297–305.

37 Bastian H (1996) Raising the standard: practice guidelines and consumer participation. *International Journal for Quality in Health Care*, **8**: 485–90.

38 Phillips KA and Bero L (1996) Improving the use of information in medical effectiveness research. *International Journal of Quality in Health Care*, **8**: 21–30.

39 Redelmeier D, Rozin P and Kahneman D (1993) Understanding patients' decisions: cognitive and emotional perspectives. *JAMA*, **270**: 72–6.

40 Fallowfield L, Hall L, Macquire G and Baum M (1990) Psychological outcomes of different treatment policies in women with early breast cancer outside a clinical trial. *BMJ*, **301**: 575–80.

41 Chewing B and Sleuth B (1996) Medication decision-making and management: a client-centred model. *Social Science and Medicine*, **42**: 389–98.

42 National Health Service Centre for Reviews and Dissemination

(1997) *Screening for prostate cancer. The evidence.* NHS CRD, University of York.

43 Katz J (1984) Why doctors don't disclose uncertainty. *The Hastings Centre Report*, February, 35–44.

44 Eddy DM (1988) Variations in clinical practice: the role of uncertainty. In: J Dowie and A Elstein (eds) *Professional Judgement. A Reader in Clinical Decision Making.* Cambridge University Press. (pp 45–59.)

45 Haynes B, Sackett D, Gray Muir J, Cook D and Guyatt G (1996) Transferring evidence from research into practice: 1. The role of clinical care research evidence in clinical decisions. *Evidence-based Medicine*, **1**: 196–7.

46 Hershey JC and Baron J (1987) Clinical reasoning and cognitive processes. *Medical Decision Making*, **7**: 203–11.

47 Baker R and Feder G (1997) Clinical guidelines: where next? *International Journal for Quality in Health Care*, **9**: 399–404.

48 Cranney M and Walley T (1996) Same information, different decisions: the influence of evidence on the management of hypertension in the elderly. *British Journal of General Practice*, **46**: 661–3.

49 Wallston K, Wallston B and de Vellis R (1978) Development of the multidimensional Health Locus of Control (MHLC) scale. *Health Education Monographs*, **6**: 160–71.

50 Degner LF and Sloan JA (1992) Decision making during serious illness: What role do patients really want to play? *Journal of Clinical Epidemiology*, **45**: 944–50.

51 Becker MH (1974) The health belief model and personal health behaviour. *Health Education Monographs*, **2**: 324–508.

52 Blanchard CG, Labrecque MS, Ruckdeschel JC and Blanchard E (1988) Information and decision-making preferences of hospitalized adult cancer patients. *Social Science in Medicine*, **27**: 1130–9.

53 Ajzen I (1985) From intentions to actions: A theory of planned behaviour. In: J Kuhl and J Beckman (eds) *Action Control: From Cognition to Behaviour.* Springer, Berlin. (pp 11–39.)

54 Schwartzer R (1992) Self efficacy in the adoption and maintenance of health behaviours: theoretical approaches and a new method. In: R Schwartzer (ed) *Self efficacy: Through Control of Action.* Hemisphere, Washington DC. (pp 217–43.)

55 Caccavo A Di and Reid F (1995) Decisional conflict in general practice: strategies of patient management. *Social Science and Medicine*, **41**: 347–53.

56 Bradley C (1992) Factors which influence the decision whether or

not to prescribe: the dilemma facing general practitioners. *British Journal of General Practice*, **42**: 454–8.

57 Ogden J (1996) *Health Psychology. A Textbook.* Open University Press, Buckingham. (p 17.)

58 Schon DA (1988) From technical rationality to reflection-in-action. In: J Dowie and A Elstein (eds) *Professional Judgement. A Reader in Clinical Decision Making.* Cambridge University Press. (pp 60–77.)

59 Hamm RM (1988) Clinical intuition and clinical analysis: expertise and the cognitive continuum. In: J Dowie and A Elstein (eds) *Professional Judgement. A Reader in Clinical Decision Making.* Cambridge University Press. (pp 78–105.)

12
Implications and futures

Richard Baker and Allen Hutchinson

The new availability of evidence-based guidelines has important implications for healthcare services. Previous chapters have shown how they can be used in commissioning services, in informing patients, and as the basis for comprehensive implementation programmes. Together, these factors signal a change in the role of health professionals. The challenge facing the health professions is to reform training to produce professionals who can not only understand and apply the evidence summarised in guidelines, but also can explain the details to patients in ways that they can use in making decisions. The effective professional user of guidelines will have to be a more, not a less, skilled practitioner.

Introduction

The previous chapters have together presented a framework for the development and use of guidelines. In simple terms, the framework proposes that guidelines should be developed systematically from good quality research evidence, but when evidence is not available expert judgement may be employed. The degree to which evidence and judgement contribute to each recommendation must be explicit, and the guidelines must be subjected to careful appraisal before they can be recommended. Because their development is complex and costly, duplication of effort is to be avoided by the production of national guidelines that may be locally adapted provided the recommendations supported by strong evidence remain intact. Tailored implementation programmes should then be used to ensure that the guidelines do lead to appropriate change in practice. Because the recommendations in up-to-date guidelines of this type can be relied on, they will also be helpful to patients and those commissioning health services. However, several issues remain unresolved, raising implications for the future use of guidelines in healthcare. In this chapter, we consider these issues and suggest how they may influence methods of developing and using guidelines in the future.

Some of the outstanding issues are shown in Box 12.1. The question of the legal implications of good quality guidelines has been thoroughly explored by Hurwitz (1998),[1] and we will not address this here, save to note his view that courts are likely to take note of, but not slavishly follow, the growing number of rigorously developed guidelines.

Box 12.1: Issues arising from the use of guidelines

- Legal implications
- Can 'systematically developed statements to assist practitioner and patient decisions' be used in commissioning?
- What are the consequences of including judgement in guideline recommendations?
- Improving implementation: do we need to reform health services *again*?
- How should we measure compliance with guidelines?
- What type of health professional, with what skills, will be required if/when guidelines are widely used?
- How do professionals develop the skills to use guidelines with patients?

Extending the role of guidelines

Current guidelines are largely developed by, and intended to meet the needs of, health professionals. However, others will inevitably wish to make use of these summaries of the best available research evidence. As we have seen (Chapter 11), there is much more to be learnt about the most acceptable and effective methods for devising and using guidelines with patients. Guidelines as they are presently formatted are only of limited help in assisting patients understand their conditions and make decisions about their care.

In contrast to the use of guidelines with individual patients, the role of commissioning places a different set of demands on guidelines. In the UK, health authorities or health boards have led commissioning, with some fundholding practices also commissioning services. However, in the future the new primary care groups will take on a greater role. Irrespective of whether they are based in health authorities or primary care, commissioners are more interested in populations than individual patients, and they need to make choices about the provision of different services. Commissioners will place importance on information about the cost-effectiveness of healthcare interventions, but individual patients will have different concerns, in particular the likelihood that the potential benefits (benefits as defined by the individual) outweigh the potential harms (similarly defined) in their own unique case.

It is not yet clear that a single guideline can meet the needs of both patients and commissioners, while at the same time assist health professionals as they make decisions. The tension between these competing demands is particularly relevant for those recommendations substantially influenced by subjective judgement (see Chapter 5), as the judgements of commissioners, professionals and patients will often differ. Thus, as the role of guidelines is extended to include patients and commissioners, methods will be needed to include judgements relevant to each group of users; perhaps different versions of the same core guideline will be needed for different users.

Implementation

The search for effective implementation methods has been relatively unrewarding. As discussed in Chapters 8 and 9, implementation is likely to be more effective when it consists of a programme of interventions designed to match local circumstances and the particular guidelines involved. Some interventions may require the reorganisation of systems of care or patterns of work. It follows that implementation cannot be achieved by health professionals alone, as generally they will not have the time or skills to design implementation programmes, nor the responsibility for health service reorganisation. Implementation is a process that must be managed, and the more effectively it is managed the more successful it is likely to be. Thus, in addition to providing information that might support commissioning, guidelines create the requirement that managers become involved in implementation. The new system of clinical governance may be regarded as an illustration of this process.[2]

A key component of implementation is the measurement of performance. Without information about compliance with the guideline concerned, assessing the need for, and monitoring the success of, implementation will be impossible. Because information is required to manage implementation, systems for monitoring performance will develop further in the next few years. There are several approaches to performance monitoring, and they bring with them a new set of issues. The performance of the health service as a whole may be monitored through the use of a few selected indicators, such as those suggested in the new National Health Service performance framework.[2] However, the success of guideline implementation requires more detailed data collection.

In order to monitor performance, choices have to be made about which aspects of care are to be assessed. In choosing measures of performance, their importance as shown by research evidence must be taken into account. It should also be possible to measure them accurately and reproducibly. Performance measures of this type are generally referred to as 'review criteria'. Review criteria have been defined as 'systematically developed statements that can be used to assess the appropriateness of specific healthcare decisions, services, and outcomes'.[3] Methods for the development of review criteria include: those that restrict criteria developed from guidelines to those aspects of care for which convincing evidence is available;[4] those that take a slightly more inclusive approach;[5] and those that employ explicit consensus procedures to account for the problem of limited evidence.[6] There is a risk that by increasing the extent to which consensus peer opinions are included during review criteria development, the eventual assessments of care may differ substantially, depending on the particular peers taking part in criteria development.[7]

Relatively little attention has been given to methods of criteria development in comparison with that given to the development of guidelines, but as monitoring of guideline implementation becomes a normal feature of healthcare, the validity and utility of criteria will be increasingly important. Monitoring is part of the process by which healthcare is managed, and the management of clinical care, rather than simply services in general, demands systems such as clinical governance. Thus, good quality clinical practice guidelines make managed care possible. It could be argued that managed care is no more than a systematic implementation programme, and that it is an illustration of the point that implementation can not be left to health professionals alone.

Professional skills

There are also issues relating to the skills needed by health professionals who are to use guidelines most effectively. On a basic level, health professionals will need to develop some familiarity with methods of guideline development and appraisal (*see* Box 12.2). The more advanced skills will include not only the ability to take part in guideline development and implementation, but also the ability to use the information in guidelines to explain to patients the findings of research. This will require highly sophisticated communication skills, built on a patient-centred foundation, but adding a new language of risk and benefit, of personal utilities and decision analyses[8] in a form that patients can understand and use in making their decisions. The new health professional, instead of being only a user of research evidence, will have

---

Box 12.2: Skills needed by health professionals

Basic

- The essentials of guideline development
  - importance of evidence
  - types of evidence
  - consensus and its significance in comparison with evidence.
- Appraisal of guidelines
  - methods of development
  - funding
  - up to date
- Implementation
  - Ability to take part in audit, educational activities, and work with team colleagues.

Advanced

- Able to participate in guideline development and implementation
- Use guidelines in consultations to inform patients and assist them make decisions. These skills will include:
  - advanced communication skills (patient-centred consulting, explaining risks and benefits in meaningful terms, identifying patients' priorities)
  - the ability to use techniques such as decision analysis.

become someone with a thorough understanding of evidence who is also able to explain in detail that evidence to patients. This implies a new relationship between professional and patient, that places greater emphasis on the provision of information, and increases the opportunity for patients, if they wish, to choose between treatments or providers.

Conclusion: futures

As clinical guidelines become absorbed into the fabric of healthcare systems, alternative futures become possible. The futures largely depend on whether guidelines are used predominantly to manage care, or whether they are used to empower patients.

In a system where the use of guidelines to manage care takes precedence, health professionals will have a minor role in implementation, and will be relatively unskilled in use of guidelines with patients. Relatively limited resources may be devoted to training and developing professionals, and the costs of care may be relatively contained. Patients are likely to be relatively dissatisfied with care. Where patient involvement predominates, professionals will be more skilled and more highly trained, but with management excluded, implementation will be less effective and costs will be higher.

In an ideal world, a balanced system would combine the best of the alternatives, and exclude the worst. If a balanced system is to be achieved, health professionals will need new and advanced skills in implementation and patient involvement, and the challenge in the next decade will be to create professionals of this type. It is perhaps surprising that by beginning to formulate clinical guidelines from good quality research evidence, the need for a new type of health professional has emerged.

References

1 Hurwitz B (1998) *Clinical Guidelines and the Law*. Radcliffe Medical Press, Oxford.
2 Secretary of State for Health (1997) *The New NHS. Modern, Dependable*. HMSO, London.
3 Field MJ and Lohr KN (eds) (1992) *Guidelines for Clinical Practice. From Development to Use*. Institute of Medicine/National Academy Press, Washington.

4 Baker R and Fraser RC (1995) The development of review criteria: linking guidelines and quality assessment. *BMJ*, **311**: 370–3.
5 Agency for Health Care Policy and Research (1995) *Using Practice Guidelines to Evaluate Quality of Care*. AHCPR/US Department of Health and Human Services, Rockville, MD.
6 Fraser GM, Pilpel D, Kosecoff J and Brook RH (1994) Effect of panel composition on appropriateness ratings. *International Journal for Quality in Health Care*, **6**: 251–5.
7 Shekelle PG, Kahan JP, Bernstein SJ, Leape LL, Kamberg CJ and Park RE (1998) The reproducibility of a method to identify the overuse and underuse of medical procedures. *NEJM* **338**: 1888–95.
8 Baker R and Feder G (1997) Clinical practice guidelines: where next? *International Journal for Quality in Health Care*, **9**: 399–404.

Index